KIDNEY CLEANSE AND DETOX DIET COOKBOOK

Simple Recipes to Boost Kidney Function and Natural Detoxification

SCOTT M. JACQUES

Copyright © 2024 Scott M. Jacques.

Table of Contents

INTRODUCTION

In the hustle and bustle of our daily lives, we often forget to pay attention to one of our body's unsung heroes the kidneys. These remarkable organs tirelessly filter waste and toxins from our blood, maintain fluid balance, and play a pivotal role in our overall health. However, we rarely pay them the attention they deserve.

Welcome to the "Kidney Cleanse and Detox Diet Cookbook." This book is your gateway to understanding, nourishing, and revitalizing your kidneys through the power of food.

Whether you're seeking to boost kidney health, manage kidney-related conditions, or simply adopt a proactive approach to well-being, this cookbook offers a holistic approach to kidney care.

Our journey begins by unraveling the intricate connection between nutrition, detoxification, and kidney function. We'll explore the science behind detox diets and delve into the nuances of kidney-friendly nutrition.

The heart of this book lies in its collection of meticulously crafted recipes. Each dish is thoughtfully designed to be low in sodium, potassium, and phosphorus, making it suitable for those with kidney concerns. These recipes not only prioritize your health but also delight your taste buds.

As you turn the pages, remember that this cookbook is more than just a compilation of recipes; it's a step toward embracing a lifestyle that honors your kidneys. Let's embark on this culinary journey together, where food becomes a catalyst for nurturing your kidneys and enhancing your well-being.

How to Use This Cookbook

To make the most of this cookbook, follow these steps:

1. Start with knowledge.

Begin by reading the introductory chapters (Chapter 1 and Chapter 2) to understand the basics of kidney health and the science of detoxification. This knowledge will provide the foundation for your journey.

2. Assess your needs.

Consider your specific goals and needs. Are you looking to enhance kidney function, manage kidney-related conditions, or simply adopt a healthier lifestyle? Understanding your objectives will help you navigate the book effectively.

3. Explore the Recipes

Dive into the heart of the book, Chapter 5, where you'll find a diverse range of kidney-friendly recipes.

Each recipe is labeled with key nutritional information, including sodium, potassium, and phosphorus content, to assist you in making informed choices.

4. Create your meal plan.

In Chapter 7, discover sample 7-day and 14-day detox plans. Use these as a starting point or customize them to fit your preferences and dietary needs. These meal plans simplify your journey to better kidney health.

5. Embrace a holistic approach.

Don't stop at the recipes alone. Chapter 8 provides valuable insights into lifestyle changes that can support kidney health. Explore hydration, exercise, and stress management tips to complement your dietary efforts.

6. Seek inspiration and support.

Read the success stories (Chapter 9) from individuals who have benefited from the kidney cleanse. Their experiences may inspire and motivate you on your own path to kidney wellness.

7. Refer to Resources

Use the appendices for additional resources, including recommended readings, websites, and frequently asked questions (Appendix A and Appendix B).

8. Get cooking and enjoy.

Finally, start preparing the delicious recipes from Chapter 5, experiment with flavors, and savor the joy of nurturing your kidneys while indulging in wholesome meals.

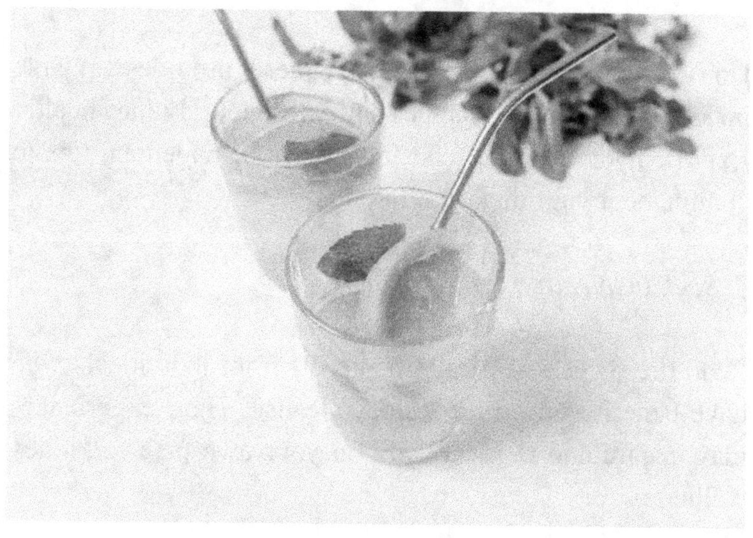

CHAPTER 1: UNDERSTANDING KIDNEY HEALTH

Our kidneys, those unassuming bean-shaped organs nestled beneath the ribcage, are the unsung heroes of our bodies. They silently perform a vital task: filtering waste and toxins from our blood, regulating electrolytes, and maintaining fluid balance. Yet we often take their relentless work for granted.

The Role of Kidneys in Your Body

To appreciate the importance of kidney health, let's first grasp their roles:

1. Filtration: Kidneys filter approximately 120–150 quarts of blood daily, removing waste and excess fluids to form urine.

2. Fluid Balance: They help maintain the balance of fluids, ensuring your body isn't overwhelmed by excess water or dehydrated.

3. Electrolyte Regulation: Kidneys manage the levels of electrolytes like sodium, potassium, and calcium, which are critical for various bodily functions.

4. Blood Pressure Control: They produce a hormone called renin, which helps regulate blood pressure.

Common Kidney Problems and Their Causes

Despite their resilience, kidneys are vulnerable to various conditions, including:

1. Chronic Kidney Disease (CKD): A gradual loss of kidney function over time, often caused by conditions like diabetes, high blood pressure, or glomerulonephritis.

2. Kidney stones: hard mineral deposits that can form in the kidneys, causing severe pain.

3. Urinary Tract Infections (UTIs): Infections that affect the urinary system, including the kidneys.

4. Polycystic Kidney Disease (PKD): A genetic disorder leading to the growth of cysts in the kidneys.

The Importance of Kidney Cleaning

Kidney cleansing is not just a trendy concept; it's a proactive step toward maintaining these essential organs. By adopting a kidney cleanse and detox diet, you can:

1. Support Kidney Function: Help your kidneys perform at their best by reducing their workload and promoting detoxification.

2. Prevent Kidney Stones: Certain foods can help prevent the formation of kidney stones.

3. Improve overall health: A healthy kidney cleanse diet can lead to better overall health and well-being.

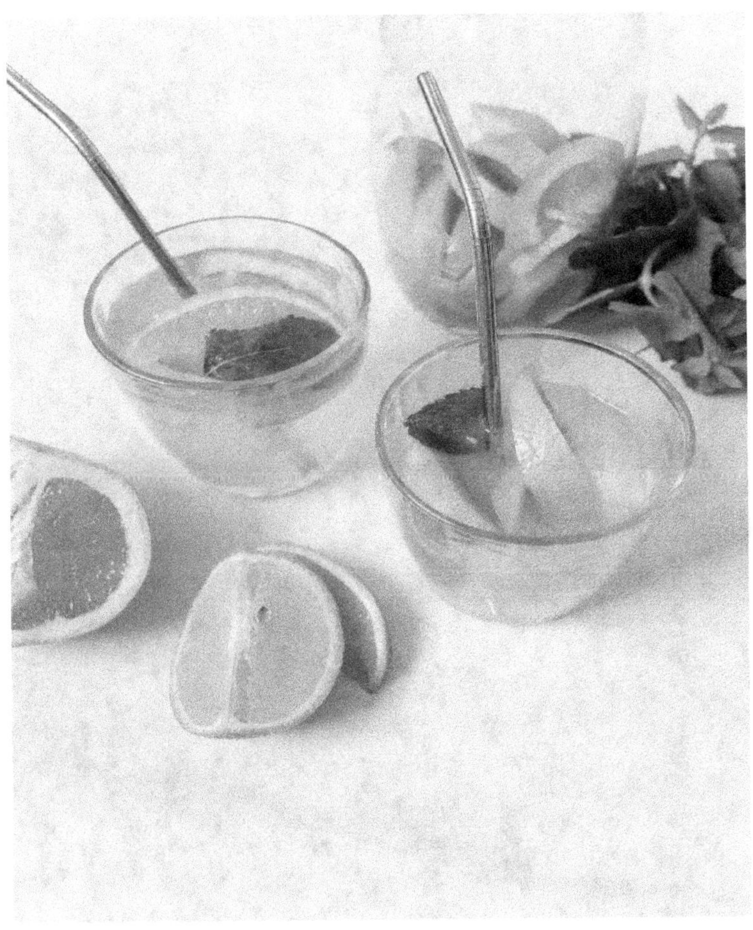

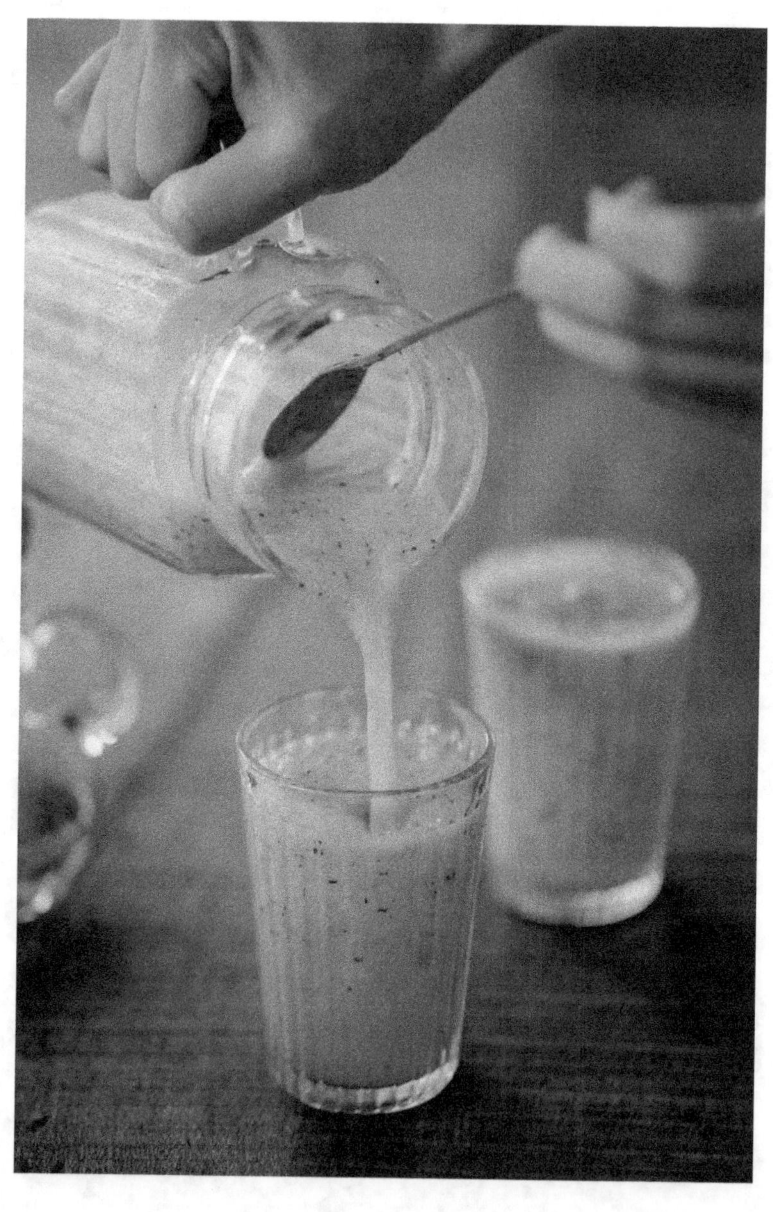

CHAPTER 2: THE SCIENCE OF DETOXIFICATION

Detoxification, a term often associated with health and wellness, is at the heart of kidney cleansing. In this chapter, we will delve into the science behind detoxification, its significance in kidney health, and the myths and facts that surround this concept.

What is Detoxification?

Detoxification is a natural, continuous process that our bodies perform to eliminate harmful substances and toxins. It involves various organs, including the liver, intestines, and, crucially, the kidneys. Here's how it works.

1. Liver Detoxification: The liver metabolizes toxins, making them water-soluble and easier to excrete.

2. Kidney Filtration: The kidneys filter these water-soluble toxins from the blood, converting them into urine.

3. Intestinal Elimination: Toxins in the gut are excreted through bowel movements.

How Detoxification Affects Kidney Health

Detoxification and kidney health are intricately linked. Here's why:

Lightening the load: A detox diet can reduce the burden on your kidneys by minimizing the intake of substances that need filtering.

Supporting Kidney Function: Certain foods and herbs can enhance kidney function and promote detoxification.

Reducing Toxins: Detox diets can help remove toxins from the body, relieving stress on the kidneys.

Balancing Electrolytes: Proper detoxification can help maintain electrolyte balance, which is essential for kidney health.

Myths and Facts about Detox Diets

Detox diets have garnered both praise and skepticism. Let's separate myths from facts:

Myth 1: Extreme fasting is necessary.
Fact: Extreme fasting can be harmful. A well-balanced detox diet is effective without extreme measures.

Myth 2: Detox Diets are a Quick Fix

Fact: Real detoxification is an ongoing process. Short-term diets may offer temporary benefits, but long-term changes are essential.

Myth 3: Detox Diets Only Involve Juicing
Fact: Detox diets encompass a variety of foods, not just juices. They focus on nutrient-dense, whole foods.

Myth 4: No Scientific Evidence
Fact: While detox diets vary, there is scientific evidence supporting their benefits, especially for specific health concerns.

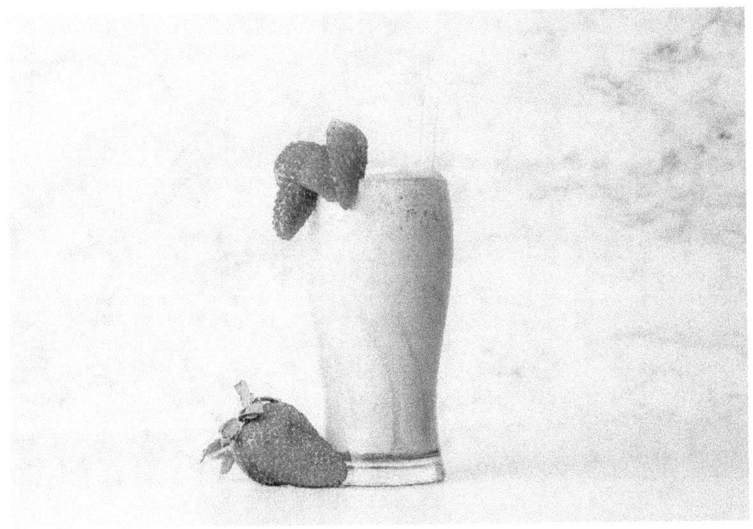

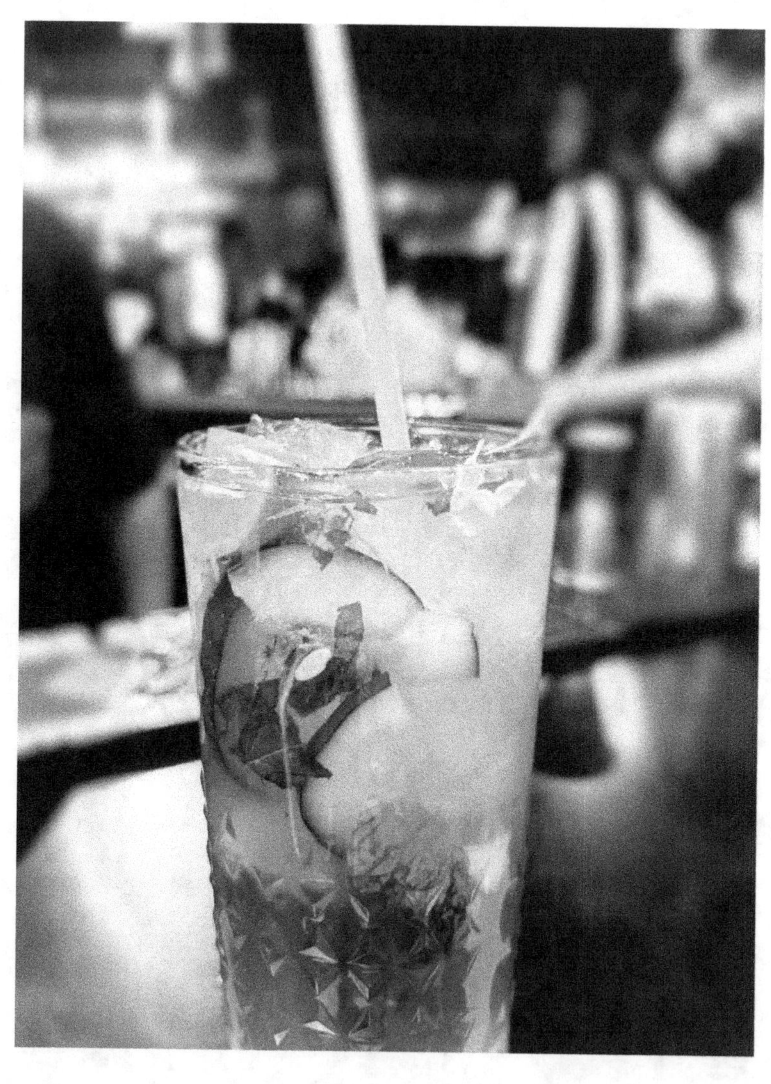

CHAPTER 3: NUTRITION AND KIDNEY HEALTH

Nutrition is the foundation of renal health. In this chapter, we will look at the critical nutrients for kidney function, foods to eat and avoid, and dietary limitations that can help you on your quest to better kidney health.

Essential Nutrients for Kidney Function

1. Protein: High-quality, lean protein sources, such as poultry, fish, and plant-based alternatives, are essential for muscle regeneration and overall health. Protein intake should be monitored because too much can strain the kidneys.

2. Sodium: Limiting sodium is critical since excess salt can raise blood pressure and strain the kidneys. Learn to read food labels and choose low-sodium options.

3. Potassium: Although potassium is necessary for heart and muscle function, an excess can be damaging to the kidneys. Reduce potassium consumption by eating low-potassium meals.

4. Phosphorus: Monitor phosphorus-rich diets, as high levels can be harmful to kidney health. Milk, legumes, and nuts are common sources.

5. Fluids: Maintaining hydration is vital for renal function. Balance your fluid intake to avoid dehydration without overburdening your kidneys.

What Foods to Eat and Avoid for Kidney Health

1. Include: Eat kidney-friendly foods like berries, leafy greens, cauliflower, and apples in your diet. They are poor in potassium and phosphorus but high in critical minerals.

2. Avoid foods that are heavy in salt, potassium, and phosphorus, such as processed meats, canned soups, and carbonated beverages. Choose dairy products with lower phosphorus levels.

Understanding Dietary Restrictions

If you have a kidney-related ailment, such as chronic kidney disease (CKD), your dietary requirements may differ. Consult a healthcare expert or qualified dietician to develop a personalized plan for your specific situation.

Special Tips for Kidney Cleansing

1. During a kidney cleanse, it is critical to limit your intake of foods that strain your kidneys. Concentrate on fresh, whole foods that promote cleansing.

2. Experiment with herbs and spices such as parsley, dandelion, and ginger, which are believed to cleanse the kidneys.

3. Gradually begin your cleanse to avoid any discomfort or adverse effects.

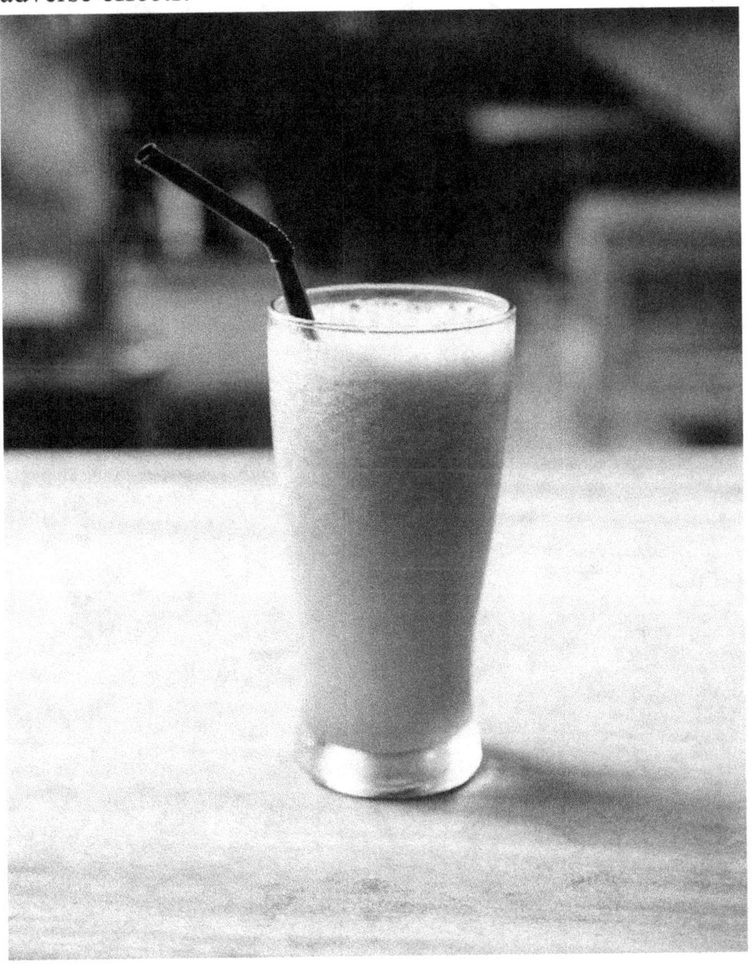

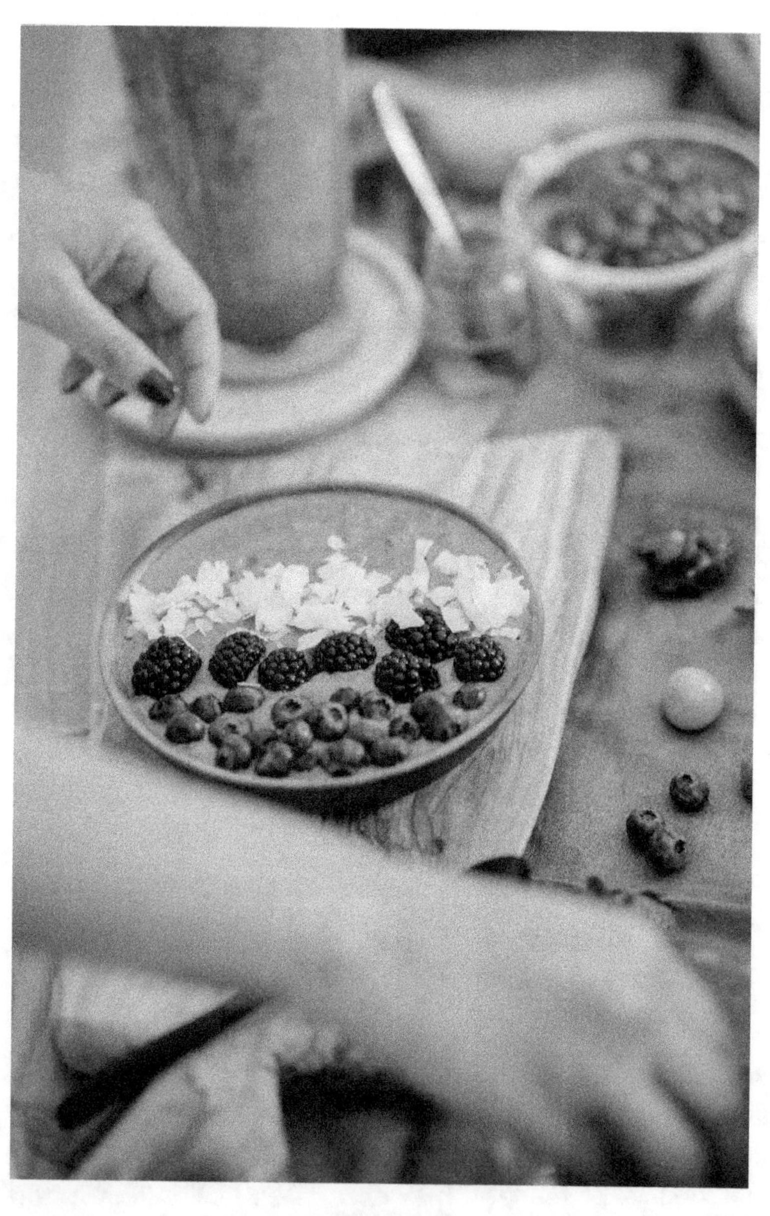

CHAPTER 4: PLANNING YOUR KIDNEY CLEANSING DIET

Starting a kidney cleanse journey involves careful planning and attention. In this chapter, we'll walk you through setting realistic goals, planning for your detox, and staying safe throughout the process.

Setting Realistic Goals

Before you start your kidney cleanse, you should clarify your goals:

1. Identify Your Goals: Do you want to improve overall kidney health, manage a specific kidney-related ailment, or simply include detoxification into your daily routine?

2. Determine Your Timeline: Decide whether you'll do a brief cleanse or incorporate kidney-friendly activities into your long-term lifestyle.

3. Consult a Healthcare Professional: If you have underlying health concerns, work with a healthcare professional or registered dietitian to develop realistic objectives that are appropriate for your circumstances.

Preparing For Your Detox

An effective kidney cleanse begins with thorough preparation.

1. Kitchen Makeover: Get rid of processed foods, high-sodium goods, and sugary beverages. Stock up on fresh vegetables, lean proteins, and kidney-friendly items.

2. Meal Planning: Plan your meals ahead of time to ensure they are consistent with your detox goals. Consider making a meal plan for the cleanse's length.

3. Shopping List: Create a shopping list based on your meal plan to prevent making last-minute unhealthy decisions.

4. Detox-Friendly Kitchen Tools: Purchase kitchen tools that will make meal preparation easier, such as a smoothie blender or a vegetable steamer.

Safety and Considerations

Safety is paramount during a kidney cleanse.

1. Monitor Your Progress: Keep a log of your meals, symptoms, and overall well-being. This can help you detect any bad responses.

2. Stay Hydrated: While adequate hydration is vital, excessive fluid consumption can strain the kidneys. For personalized advice, consult with your healthcare physician.

3. Listen to Your Body: If you are experiencing discomfort or strange symptoms, seek medical attention right once.

4. Gradual Transition: Start your kidney cleanse gradually to limit the possibility of unwanted effects.

5. Supplements and Herbs: If you're thinking about using supplements or herbs to help with your cleanse, talk to your doctor first to make sure they're safe and right for you.

Setting reasonable goals, planning ahead of time, and prioritizing safety will prepare you well for your kidney cleanse journey. In the next chapters, we'll look at a selection of delectable meals that will help your kidneys while also improving your general health.

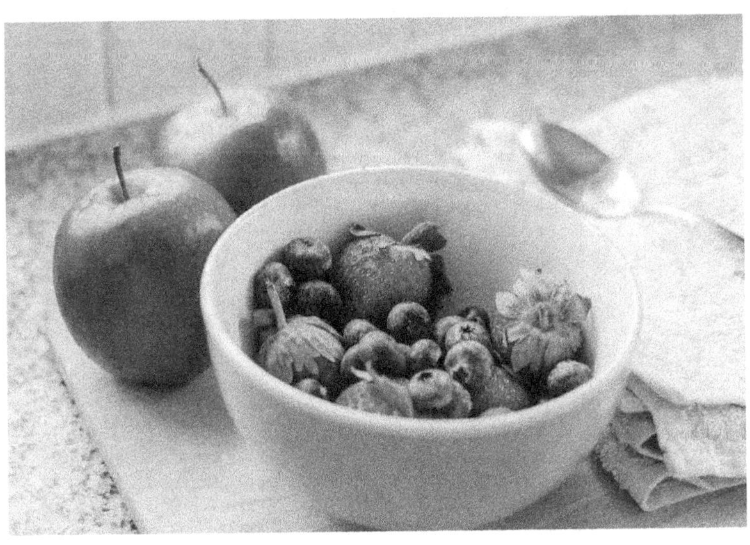

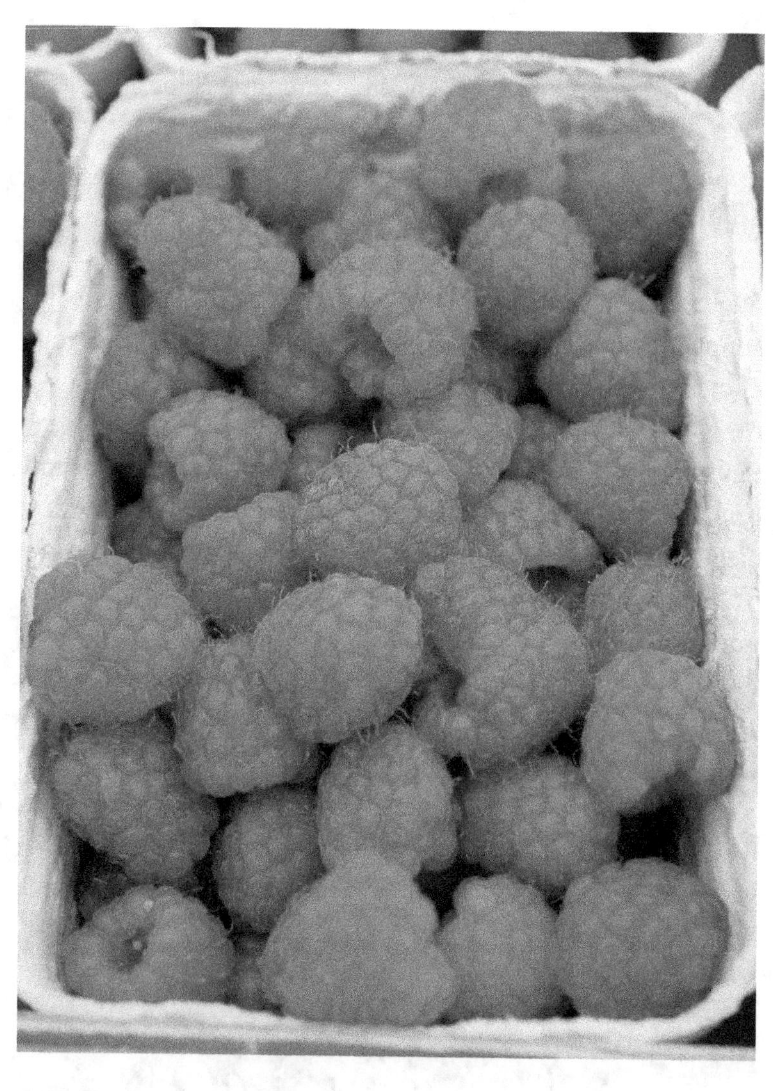

CHAPTER 5: DETOXIFYING RECIPES

Morning Starters and Smoothies

1. Green Cleansing Smoothie

Ingredients:

- 1 cup of fresh spinach.
- 1/2 green apple, cut
- 1/2 banana.
- 1/2 cucumber.
- 1 tablespoon of chia seeds.
- 1 cup of almond milk.
- 1 teaspoon of honey (optional)

Instructions:

1. Use a blender to combine every ingredient.

2. Blend until smooth or set.

Preparation time: 5 minutes

Nutritional value (approx):

- Calories: 180

- Protein: 3g
- Carbohydrate: 35g
- Fat: 4g
- Fiber: 6g

2. Berry Blast Breakfast Bowl

Ingredients:

- 1/2 cup of rolled oats.
- 1 cup of almond milk.
- 1/2 cup of mixed berries (i.e blueberries, strawberries, and raspberries).
- 1 tablespoon of sliced almonds.
- 1 teaspoon of honey or maple syrup.
- 1 tablespoon of flaxseeds.

Instructions:

1. Soak the oats in almond milk overnight.

2. In the morning, top with a mix of berries, almonds, honey, and flax seeds.

Preparation time is overnight (plus 5 minutes in the morning).

Nutritional value (approx):

- Calories: 300
- Protein: 8g
- Carbohydrate: 50g
- Fat: 9g
- Fiber: 7g

3. Detoxifying Citrus Elixir

Ingredients:

- 1 cup of water and lemon juice.
- 1 teaspoon of grated ginger.
- 1 tablespoon of apple cider vinegar.
- 1 teaspoon of honey.

Instructions:

1. Combine all of the ingredients in a glass and whisk thoroughly.

Preparation time: 5 minutes

Nutritional value (approx):

- Calories: 40
- Protein: 0g
- Carbohydrate: 10g
- Fat: 0g

- Fiber: 0g

4. Creamy Banana Oatmeal

Ingredients:

- 1/2 cup of rolled oats.
- 1 cup of almond milk.
- 1 ripe, mashed banana
- 1/2 teaspoon of cinnamon.
- 1 tablespoon of honey or maple syrup.

Instructions:

1. Heat the oats and almond milk in a saucepan over medium heat.

2. Stir in the mashed banana, cinnamon, and honey.

3. Cook to the desired consistency.

Preparation time: 5 minutes
Cooking time: 10 minutes.

Nutritional value (approx):

- Calories: 320
- Protein: 6g

- Carbohydrate: 65g
- Fat: 6g
- Fiber: 7g

5. Refreshing Mint Cooler

Ingredients:

- 1 cup of water.
- A handful of fresh mint leaves.
- 1 lime juice
- 1 teaspoon of honey (optional)
- Ice cubes

Instructions:

1. Muddle the mint leaves with water.

2. Add the lime juice and honey, and combine thoroughly.

3. Serve with ice cubes.

Preparation time: 5 minutes

Nutritional value (approx):

- Calories: 20
- Protein: 0g

- Carbohydrate: 5g
- Fat: 0g
- Fiber: 0g

6. Pineapple and Kale Smoothie

Ingredients:

- 1 cup of chopped kale with stems removed.
- 1 cup of frozen pineapple pieces.
- 1/2 banana.
- 1 cup of coconut water.
- 1 tablespoon of flaxseeds.

Instructions:

1. Use a blender to combine every ingredient.

2. Blend until smooth and creamy.

Preparation time: 5 minutes

Nutritional value (approx):

- Calories: 200
- Protein: 4g
- Carbs: 47g
- Fat: 4g

- Fiber: 5g

7. Chia Pudding Parfait

Ingredients:

- 3 tablespoons of chia seeds.
- 1 cup of almond milk.
- 1/2 teaspoon of vanilla extract.
- 1 tablespoon of maple syrup.
- 1/2 cup of fresh berries.
- 1/4 cup of granola.

Instructions:

1. Combine chia seeds, almond milk, vanilla extract, and maple syrup in a bowl.

2. Refrigerate overnight.

3. Prior to serving, layer the chia pudding with berries and granola.

Preparation time is overnight (plus 5 minutes in the morning).

Nutritional value (approx):

- Calories: 310
- Protein: 8g
- Carbs: 44g
- Fat: 12g
- Fiber: 14g

8. Turmeric Golden Milk Smoothie

Ingredients:

- 1 cup of almond milk.
- 1/2 banana.
- 1/2 teaspoon of ground turmeric.
- 1/4 teaspoon of ground ginger.
- A pinch of black pepper.
- 1 tablespoon of honey.

Instructions:

1. Combine all of the ingredients and blend until smooth.

Preparation time: 5 minutes

Nutritional value (approx):

- Calories: 150
- Protein: 2g
- Carbohydrate: 32g

- Fat: 3g
- Fiber: 3g

9. Protein-Rich Quinoa Bowl

Ingredients:

- 1/2 cup of cooked quinoa.
- 1/4 cup black beans.
- 1/4 cup corn.
- 1/4 avocado, sliced
- 1/2 tomato, diced
- 1 tablespoon olive oil
- 1 lime juice
- Salt and pepper

Instructions:

1. In a bowl, combine the quinoa, black beans, corn, avocado, and tomato.

2. Pour in some lime juice and olive oil.

3. Season with salt and pepper.

Preparation time: 10 minutes
Cooking time: 15 minutes for quinoa.

Nutritional value (approx):

- Calories: 340
- Protein: 10g
- Carbs: 45g
- Fat: 15g
- Fiber: 8g

10. Mango Tango Smoothie

Ingredients:

- 1 cup of frozen mango chunks.
- 1/2 banana.
- 1/2 cup of orange juice.
- 1/2 cup of Greek yogurt.
- 1 tablespoon of honey.

Instructions:

1. Combine all of the ingredients and blend until smooth.

Preparation time: 5 minutes

Nutritional value (approx):

- Calories: 250
- Protein: 8g

- Carbs: 55g
- Fat: 1g
- Fiber: 3g

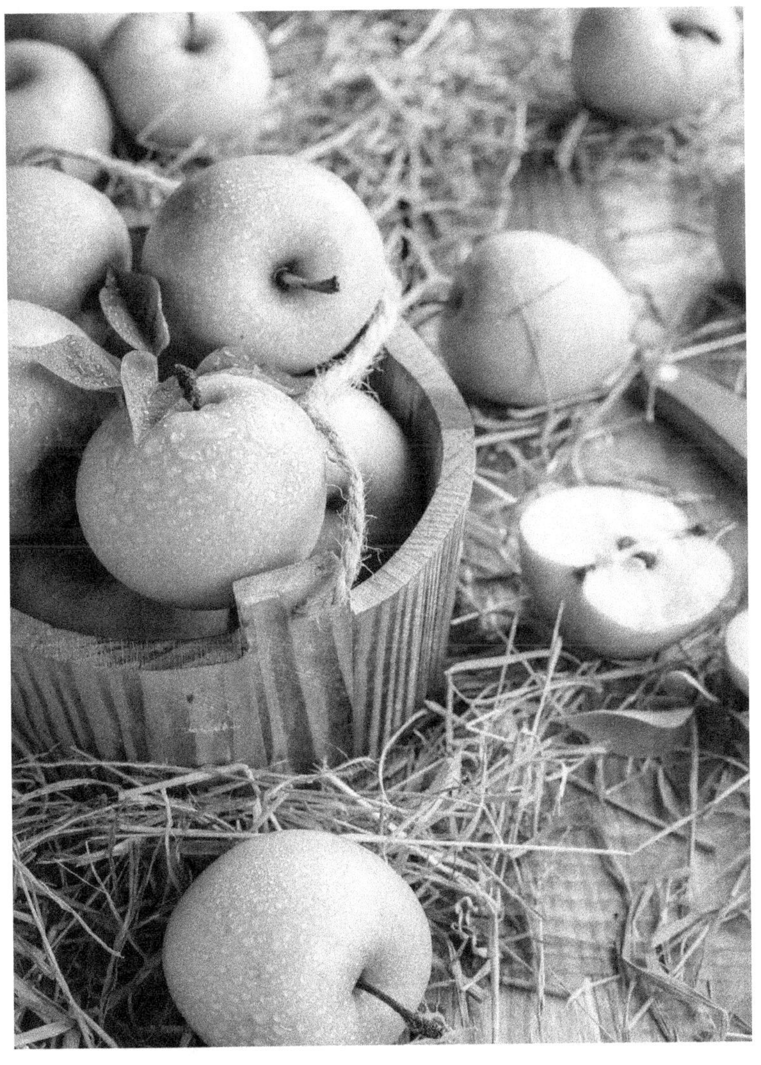

Nourishing Breakfasts

11. Vegetable Omelet

Ingredients:

- 2 eggs
- 1/4 cup of chopped bell peppers.
- 1/4 cup of chopped spinach.
- 2 tablespoons of diced onions
- 1 tablespoon of olive oil.
- Salt and pepper
- 1 tablespoon of shredded cheese (optional).

Instructions:

1. In a mixing basin, beat the eggs until smooth or set. Add some salt and pepper.

2. In a baking pan, heat olive oil and cook the onions, bell peppers and spinach until tender.

3. Pour the eggs over the vegetables, heat again until set. Add cheese if desired.
4. Serve.

Preparation time: 5 minutes
Cooking time: 10 minutes.

Nutritional value (approx):

- Calories: 250
- Protein: 14g
- Carbs: 6g
- Fat: 19g
- Fiber: 1g

12. Avocado Toast with Poached Eggs

Ingredients:

- 1 slice of whole grain bread.
- 1/2 ripe of avocado.
- 1 egg
- Salt and pepper
- Toppings (i.e red pepper flakes and chia seeds optional)

Instructions:

1. Toast the bread. Mash the avocado onto the toasted bread.

2. Poach the egg in simmering water and set it on top of the avocado.

3. Season with salt, pepper and optional toppings.

4. Serve.

Preparation time: 5 minutes
Cooking time: 10 minutes.

Nutritional value (approx):

- Calories: 300
- Protein: 12g
- Carbs: 30g
- Fat: 17g
- Fiber: 7g

13. Steel-Cut Oatmeal with Berries

Ingredients:

- 1/4 cup of steel-cut oats.
- 1 cup of water or milk.
- 1/2 cup of mixed berries.
- 1 tablespoon of honey or maple syrup.
- 1 tablespoon of chia seeds (optional).

Instructions:

1. Cook the oats in water or milk according to package directions.

2. Top with the berries, sweetener and chia seeds.

3. Serve.

Preparation time: 5 minutes
Cooking time: 20-30 minutes.

Nutritional value (approx):

- Calories: 220
- Protein: 6g
- Carbohydrate: 40g
- Fat: 5g
- Fiber: 6g

14. Greek Yogurt Parfait

Ingredients:

- 1 cup of Greek yogurt.
- 1/2 cup of granola.
- 1/2 cup of mixed berries.
- 1 tablespoon of honey or maple syrup.

Instructions:

1. In a glass or dish, mix Greek yogurt, granola and berries.

2. Drizzle with honey or syrup.

3. Serve.

Preparation time: 5 minutes

Nutritional value (approx):

- Calories: 350
- Protein: 20g
- Carbs: 45g
- Fat: 10g
- Fiber: 4g

15. Smoked Salmon with Scrambled Eggs

Ingredients:

- 2 eggs
- 2 ounces smoked salmon, sliced.
- 1 tablespoon of cream cheese
- 1 tablespoon chives, chopped
- 1 teaspoon olive oil.
- Salt and pepper

Instructions:

1. Combine the eggs with salt and pepper.

2. Heat the oil in a baking pan and scramble the eggs to your satisfaction.

3. Stir in the cream cheese and fish.

4. Top with chives and serve.

Preparation time: 5 minutes
Cooking time: 5 minutes.

Nutritional value (approx):

- Calories: 300
- Protein: 23g
- Carbs: 2g
- Fat: 22g
- Fiber: 0g

16. Sweet Potato Hash

Ingredients:

- 1 large sweet potato, peeled and chopped
- 1/2 red bell pepper, diced.
- 1/2 onion, diced.
- 2 garlic cloves, minced
- 2 tablespoons of olive oil.
- Salt and pepper

- 2 eggs (optional, as topping)

Instructions:

1. In a baking pan, heat the olive oil.

2. Cook the onion and garlic until soft or set.

3. Add the sliced sweet potatoes and bell peppers.

4. Cook until the potatoes are soft or set.

5. Optional: top with fried or poached eggs

Preparation time: 10 minutes
Cooking time: 20 minutes.

Nutritional Value (approx, excluding eggs):

- Calories: 250
- Protein: 3g
- Carbohydrate: 35g
- Fat: 11g
- Fiber: 5g

17. Quinoa Breakfast Bowl

Ingredients:

- 1/2 cup of cooked quinoa.
- 1/2 banana, cut.
- 1/4 cup of chopped almonds.
- 1/4 cup of blueberries.
- 1 tablespoon of honey or maple syrup.
- 1/2 cup of almond milk.

Instructions:

1. In a mixing bowl, combine cooked quinoa and almond milk.

2. Garnish with banana slices, almonds, blueberries.

3. Drizzle with honey or syrup.

4. Serve.

Preparation Time: 5 minutes (if the quinoa is precooked).

Nutritional value (approx):

- Calories: 350
- Protein: 9g
- Carbs: 55g
- Fat: 12g
- Fiber: 7g

18. Blueberry Pancakes

Ingredients:

- 1 cup of all-purpose flour
- 1 tablespoon of sugar.
- 1 teaspoon of baking powder.
- 1/2 teaspoon of baking soda.
- 1/4 teaspoon of salt.
- 1 egg
- 3/4 cup of buttermilk.
- 1/4 cup of blueberries.
- 1 tablespoon of butter for cooking.

Instructions:

1. In a mixing bowl, combine the flour, sugar, baking powder, baking soda and salt.

2. In another mixing bowl, combine the egg and buttermilk. Mix into the dry ingredients thoroughly.

3. Gently fold in the blueberries.

4. Cook the pancakes in a greased skillet until golden or set.

5. Serve.

Preparation time: 10 minutes

Cooking time: 10 minutes.

Nutritional value (per pancake, yields approximately 8):

- Calories: 100
- Protein: 3g
- Carbohydrate: 15g
- Fat: 3g
- Fiber: 1g

19. Spinach and Mushroom Frittata

Ingredients:

- 4 eggs
- 1 cup of spinach, chopped
- 1/2 cup of sliced mushrooms.
- 1/4 cup of onion, chopped
- 1/4 cup of cheese, grated
- 1 tablespoon of olive oil.
- Salt and pepper

Instructions:

1. Preheat the oven to 350°F (175°C).

2. Cook the onions, mushrooms and spinach in olive oil and set aside.

3. Whisk the eggs, cheese, salt, and pepper then combine with cooked vegetables.

4. Place the mixture in a baking pan.

5. Bake until the eggs are set.

Preparation time: 10 minutes
Cooking time: 20 minutes.

Nutritional value (per serving: serve 4):

- Calories: 160
- Protein: 10g
- Carbohydrate: 4g
- Fat: 12g
- Fiber: 1g

20. Homemade Muesli

Ingredients:

- 2 cups of rolled oats.
- 1/2 cup of raisins.
- 1/2 cup of chopped almonds.

- 1/4 cup of sunflower seeds.
- 1/4 cup of dried cranberries.
- 1/4 teaspoon of cinnamon.
- Almond milk or yogurt to serve.

Instructions:

1. In a large basin, combine all the dry ingredients.

2. Store in an airtight container.

3. Serve alongside almond milk or yogurt.

Preparation time: 10 minutes

Nutritional value (per 1/2 cup portion, excluding milk and yogurt):

- Calories: 200
- Protein: 6g
- Carbs: 30g
- Fat: 8g
- Fiber: 4g

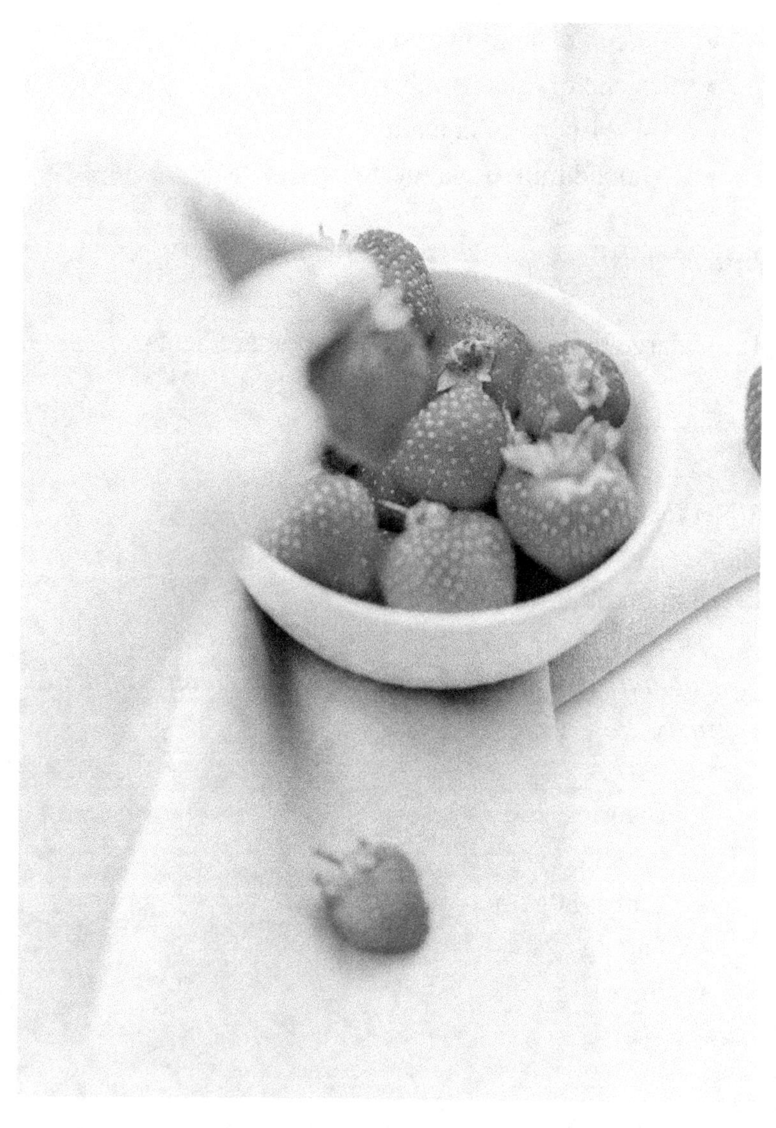

Light Meals and Salads

21. Cucumber Kidney Cleanse Salad

Ingredients:

- 2 cucumbers
- 1/4 mug red onion
- 1/4 mug apple cider vinegar
- 2 soupspoons olive oil
- 1 teaspoon honey
- 1/4 mug fresh dill
- Seasoning

Preparation Time: 15 minutes
Cooking Time: 0 minutes

Instructions:

1. Cut the cucumbers and red onion into thin slices.

2. Mix the apple cider vinegar, olive oil, honey and seasoning.

3. Toss cucumbers, onion, and dill with the dressing.

4. Chill before serving.

Nutritional Value:

- Calories: 120
- Fat: 7g
- Sodium: 10 mg
- Carbs: 13g
- Protein: 1g.

22. Kidney Beans with Quinoa Salad

Ingredients:

- 1 mug cooked quinoa
- 1 mug cooked kidney beans
- 1 minced bell pepper
- 1/4 mug diced parsley
- 2 soupspoons lemon juice,
- 1 teaspoon olive oil
- Seasoning

Preparation Time: 10 minutes
Cooking Time: 15 minutes (for quinoa)

Instructions:

1. In a mixing dish, combine the cooked quinoa and kidney beans.

2. Add minced bell pepper and diced parsley.

3. Dress with lemon juice, olive oil, salt and pepper.

4. Mix completely.

Nutritional Value:

- Calories: 200
- Fat: 5g
- Sodium: 15 mg
- Carbohydrates: 30g
- Protein: 9g.

23. Apple and Walnut Spinach Salad

Ingredients:

- 3 mugs baby spinach
- 1 sliced apple
- 1/4 mug walnuts
- 2 teaspoons of balsamic vinegar
- 1 teaspoon olive oil
- Seasoning

Preparation Time: 10 minutes
Cooking Time: 0 minute

Instructions:

1. In a large coliseum, mix the spinach, apple pieces, and walnuts.

2. Mizzle with balsamic vinegar and olive oil.

3. Season with salt and pepper.

Nutritional Value:

- Calories: 150
- Fat: 9g
- Sodium: 25mg
- Carbs: 16g
- Protein: 3g

24. Avocado and Tomato Salad

Ingredients:

- 2 ripe avocados,
- 2 minced tomatoes,
- 1/4 mug diced red onion,
- 2 soupspoons lime juice,
- 1 teaspoon olive oil
- Salt and pepper

Preparation Time: 10 minutes

Cooking Time: 0 minute

Instructions:

1. Cube avocados and sliced tomatoes.

2. In a mixing coliseum, blend avocados, tomatoes, and red onion.

3. Mizzle with lime juice and olive oil.

4. Season with salt and pepper.

Nutritional Value:

- Calories: 220
- Fat: 17g
- Sodium: 10mg
- Carbs: 18g
- Protein: 3g

25. Beetroot and Goat Cheese Salad

Ingredients:

- 3 cooked beetroots,
- 1/4 mug crumbled goat cheese

- 2 mugs arugula,
- 2 teaspoons olive oil
- 1 teaspoon balsamic glaze
- Salt and pepper

Preparation Time: 10 minutes
Cooking Time: 0 minute

Instructions:

1. Slice beetroots thinly.

2. In a serving plate, blend arugula, sliced beetroot, and crumbled goat cheese.

3. Mizzle with olive oil and a balsamic glaze.

4. Season with salt and pepper.

Nutritional value:

- Calories: 180
- Fat: 8g
- Sodium: 130mg
- Carbs: 13g
- Protein: 6g

26. Carrot and Ginger Soup

Ingredients:

- 4 mugs diced carrots,
- 1 teaspoon grated ginger,
- 1 diced onion,
- 4 mugs vegetable broth,
- 1 teaspoon olive oil
- Salt and pepper

Preparation time: 10 minutes
Cooking time: 30 minutes

Instructions:

1. Cook onion and ginger in olive oil till tender or set.

2. Mix carrots and vegetable broth.

3. Bring to a boil, also reduce heat and allow it to poach until the carrots are soft.

4. Mix until smooth.

5. Season with salt and pepper.

Nutritional value:

- Calories: 110
- Fat: 4g
- Sodium: 50mg
- Carbs: 17g
- Protein: 2g

27. Lemon Garlic Kale Salad

Ingredients:

- 4 mugs diced kale,
- 2 soupspoons lemon juice,
- 1 teaspoon olive oil
- 1 diced garlic clove,
- Salt and pepper
- 1/4 mug sliced almonds.

Preparation Time: 15 minutes
Cooking Time: 0 minute

Instructions:

1. Mix kale with lemon juice, olive oil, garlic, salt and pepper until tender.

2. Before serving, garnish with sliced almonds.

Nutritional value:

- Calories: 140
- Fat: 9g
- Sodium: 30mg
- Carbs: 12g
- Protein: 5g

28. Asparagus and Egg Salad

Ingredients:

- 2 mugs diced asparagus,
- 4 cooked eggs,
- 2 teaspoons Dijon mustard,
- 1 teaspoon olive oil,
- 1 teaspoon lemon juice,
- Salt and pepper

Preparation Time: 10 minutes
Cooking Time: 10 minutes

Instructions:

1. Boil the asparagus until tender-crisp.

2. Slice the boiled eggs.

3. To make the dressing, blend Dijon mustard, olive oil, and lemon juice.

4. Mix the asparagus, eggs, and dressing.

5. Season with salt and pepper.

Nutritional value:

- Calories: 160
- Fat: 11g
- Sodium: 210 mg
- Carbs: 4g
- Protein: 12g

29. Watermelon and Feta Salad

Ingredients:

- 4 mugs cubed watermelon
- 1/2 mug crumbled feta cheese
- 1/4 mug fresh mint leaves
- 2 teaspoons balsamic glaze.

Preparation Time: 10 minutes
Cooking Time: 0 minute

Instructions:

1. Mix watermelon, feta cheese, and mint leaves in a clean mixing coliseum.

2. Mizzle with balsamic glaze before serving.

Nutritional value:

- Calories: 120
- Fat: 5g
- Sodium: 180 mg
- Carbs: 17g
- Protein: 4g

30. Broccoli and Chickpea Salad

Ingredients:

- 2 mugs diced broccoli,
- 1 mug cooked chickpeas,
- 1 minced red bell pepper,
- 1/4 mug diced red onion,
- 2 soupspoons lemon juice,
- 1 teaspoon olive oil
- Salt and peppers

Preparation Time: 15 minutes
Cooking Time: 0 minute

Instructions:

1. Mix broccoli, chickpeas, bell pepper, and onion in a large mixing coliseum.

2. Dress with lemon juice and olive oil.

3. Season with salt and pepper.

Nutritional value:

- Calories: 150
- Fat: 5g
- Sodium: 30 mg
- Carbs: 22g
- Protein: 7g

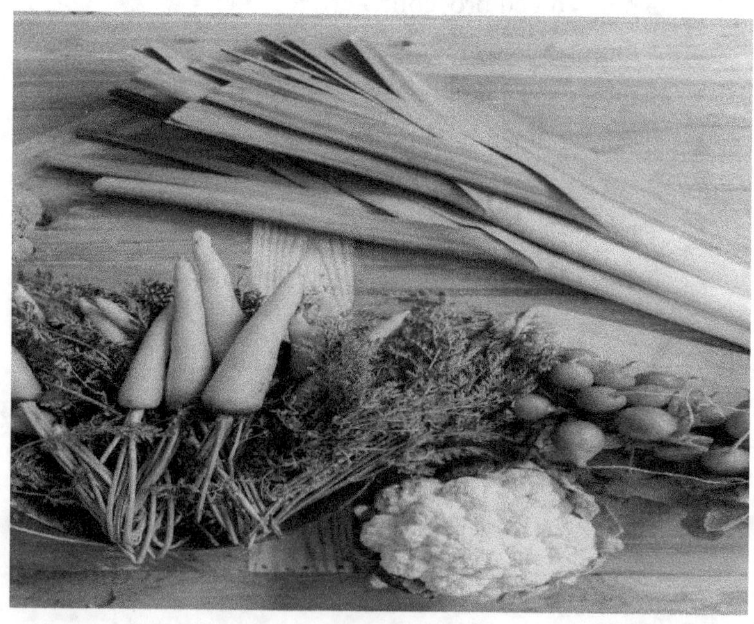

Healthy Soups and Stews

31. Minestrone Soup

Ingredients:

- 1 teaspoon of olive.
- 1 onion, diced
- 2 carrots, minced
- 2 celery stalks, minced
- 3 garlic cloves, diced
- 1 zucchini, minced
- 1 mug of green beans, trimmed and cut into 1/2-inch pieces.
- 1 can (14.5 ounces) minced tomatoes
- 4 mugs veggie broth.
- 1 can (15 oz) of cannellini beans, dried and rinsed
- 1/2 mug tiny pasta (i.e ditalini)
- 1 tablespoon of dried oregano.
- 1 tablespoon dried basil.
- Salt and pepper.
- 1/4 mug of grated Parmesan cheese (optional for serving)
- 2 soupspoons freshly diced parsley (for garnish).

Instructions:

1. Toast the olive oil in a big pot over medium heat.

2. Cook the onion, carrots, celery, and garlic until softened for 5 minutes.

3. Mix the zucchini, green beans, minced tomatoes, and vegetable broth, also bring to a boil.

4. Mix in the cannellini beans, pasta, oregano and basil.

5. Reduce the heat and cook the pasta for about 10-15 minutes.

6. Season with salt and pepper.

7. Top with Parmesan cheese and fresh parsley.

8. Serve.

Preparation time: 15 minutes
Cooking time: 30 minutes

Nutritional value (per serving):

- Calories: 200
- Fat: 3g
- Carbs: 35g
- Protein: 9g
- Fiber: 8g

32. Sweet Potato and Lentil Stew

Ingredients:

- 1 teaspoon of olive oil
- 1 onion, diced
- 2 garlic cloves, diced
- 1 large sweet potato, hulled and diced
- 1 mug of red lentils, washed.
- 4 mugs of veggie broth.
- 1 tablespoon of ground cumin.
- 1 tablespoon of smoked paprika.
- Salt and pepper.
- Fresh cilantro, diced (to garnish)

Instructions

1. Toast the olive oil in a big pot over medium heat.

2. Cook the onion and garlic until softened, about 5 minutes.

3. Mix the sweet potato, red lentils, vegetable broth, cumin, and smoky paprika.

4. Bring to a boil, also drop heat and cover until lentils and sweet potato are cooked, about 20- 25 minutes.

5. Season with salt and pepper.

6. Serve hot, garnished with diced cilantro.

Preparation time: 10 minutes
Cooking time: 30 minutes

Nutritional value (per serving):

- Calories: 240
- Fat: 3g
- Carbs: 42g
- Protein: 12g
- Fiber: 19g

33. Chicken and Vegetable Soup

Ingredients:

- 1 teaspoon of olive oil
- 1 onion, diced
- 2 carrots, minced
- 2 celery stalks, minced
- 2 garlic cloves diced
- 1 pound of skinless, boneless chicken breast, sliced into small pieces.
- 6 mugs of chicken broth.
- 1 mug of frozen peas.
- 1 tablespoon of dried thyme.
- Salt and pepper.

- Fresh parsley, diced (to garnish)

Instructions:

1. Toast the olive oil in a big pot over medium heat.

2. Cook the onion, carrots, celery, and garlic until softened, about 5 minutes.

3. Cook the chicken until no longer pink, about 5- 7 minutes.

4. Pour in the chicken broth and heat to a boil. Reduce the heat to simmer for 15 minutes.

5. Stir in the peas and thyme, simmer for a further 5 minutes.

6. Season with salt and pepper.

7. Serve hot and garnish with fresh parsley.

Preparation time: 15 minutes
Cooking time: 30 minutes

Nutritional value (per serving):

- Calories: 220
- Fat: 4g
- Carbs: 15g
- Protein: 30g

- Fiber: 3g

34. Tomato Basil Soup

Ingredients:

- 2 soupspoons of olive oil.
- 1 onion, diced
- 2 cloves of garlic, diced
- 2 cans (14.5 oz each), minced tomatoes, undrained
- 4 mugs of veggie broth
- 1/2 mug of diced fresh basil leaves.
- Salt and pepper.
- 1/2 mug heavy cream (optional)

Instructions:

1. Toast the olive oil in a big pot over medium heat.

2. Cook the onion and garlic until softened, about 5 minutes.
3. Mix the minced tomatoes (with juice) and vegetable broth.

4. Bring to a boil, then reduce the heat and simmer for at least 15 minutes.

5. Add fresh basil and season with salt and pepper.

6. With an absorption blender, purée the haze until smooth.

7. Stir in the heavy cream and heat until completely combined.

8. Serve hot.

Preparation time: 10 minutes
Cooking time: 25 minutes

Nutritional value (per serving):

- Calories (without cream): 150
- Fat: 10g
- Carbs: 13g
- Protein: 2g
- Fiber: 3g

35. Bean and Kale Soup

Ingredients:

- 1 teaspoon of olive oil
- 1 onion, diced
- 2 garlic cloves, diced
- 1 can (15 oz) of cannellini beans, dried and rinsed
- 4 mugs veggie broth.
- 4 mugs diced kale.
- 1 tablespoon dried thyme.
- Salt and pepper

- Grated parmesan cheese (optional for serving)

Instructions:

1. Toast the olive oil in a big pot over medium heat.

2. Cook the onion and garlic until softened for at least 5 minutes.

3. Mix the cannellini beans, vegetable broth, and kale.

4. Bring to a boil, also reduce heat and simmer for 10 minutes, or until the kale is soft.

5. Add thyme, salt and pepper.

6. Garnish with grated Parmesan cheese if preferred and serve hot.

Preparation time: 10 minutes
Cooking time: 20 minutes

Nutritional value (per serving):

- Calories: 180
- Fat: 3g
- Carbs: 30g
- Protein: 10g
- Fiber: 8g

36. Spicy Thai Coconut Soup

Ingredients:

- 1 teaspoon of coconut oil
- 1 onion, diced
- 2 garlic cloves, diced
- 1 teaspoon of ginger, grated
- 1 lemongrass stalk, diced
- 2 soupspoons of red curry paste.
- 4 mugs of chicken or vegetarian broth.
- 1 can (14 ounces) of coconut milk
- 1 pound of thinly sliced chicken breast (forget chicken if vegetarian).
- 1 mug of sliced mushrooms
- 2 teaspoons of fish sauce (vegetarian can use soy sauce rather).
- 1 teaspoon of sugar.
- Juice of 1 lime
- 1/4 mug of fresh cilantro, diced
- Salt.

Instructions:

1. Preheat the coconut oil in a saucepan over medium heat.

2. Cook onion, garlic, grated ginger, and lemongrass until fragrant, about 2 minutes.

3. Stir in the red curry paste, then add the broth and coconut milk. Bring to a boil.

4. Combine the chicken (if using), mushrooms, fish sauce and sugar.

5. Cook for 15- 20 minutes, or until the chicken is completely cooked.

6. Add the lime juice, then season with salt and stir.

7. Serve hot and sprinkle with cilantro.

Preparation time: 10 minutes
Cooking time: 30 minutes

Nutritional value (per serving):

- Calories: 310
- Fat: 19g
- Carbs: 9g
- Protein: 28g
- Fiber: 1g

37. Black-eye Pea Stew

Ingredients:

- 1 teaspoon of olive oil
- 1 onion, diced
- 3 diced garlic cloves
- 1 diced bell pepper
- 2 mugs of black- eyed peas soaked and drained overnight.
- 4 mugs of veggie broth.
- 1 can (14.5 ounces) of minced tomatoes
- 1 tablespoon of smoked paprika.
- 1 tablespoon of cumin.
- Salt and pepper.
- 2 mugs of kale, diced

Instructions:

1. In a large pot, toast the olive oil over medium heat.

2. Cook for about 5 minutes, or until the onion, garlic and bell pepper soften.

3. Mix the black-eyed peas, vegetable broth, minced tomatoes, smoked paprika and cumin.

4. Bring to a boil, then reduce the heat and simmer for 1 hour, or until the peas are cooked.

5. Season with salt and pepper.

6. Stir in the kale and cook for 5 minutes, or until wilted.

7. Serve hot.

Preparation time: 10 minutes (including soaking).
Cooking time: 1 hour 10 minutes.

Nutritional value (per serving):

- Calories: 210
- Fat: 3g
- Carbs: 36g
- Protein: 12g
- Fiber: 9g

38. Butternut Squash Soup

Ingredients:

- 2 soupspoons of olive oil
- 1 onion, diced
- 1 butternut squash (about 2 lbs) peeled, seeded and cubed
- 4 mugs of veggie broth.
- 1/2 tablespoon of nutmeg.
- Salt and pepper.
- 1/2 mug of heavy cream (optional for vegan, forget or substitute coconut milk)

Instructions:

1. In a large pot, toast the olive oil over medium heat.

2. Add the onion and simmer for about 5 minutes, or until transparent.

3. Mix butternut squash and vegetable broth.

4. Bring to a boil, then reduce the heat and simmer for 20 minutes, or until the squash is soft.

5. Puree the haze with an absorption blender or in batches in a blender.

6. Season the mixture with nutmeg, salt, and pepper.

7. Stir in the heavy cream and heat well, If using.

8. Serve hot.

Preparation time: 15 minutes
Cooking time: 25 minutes

Nutritional value (per serving):

- Calories (without cream): 180
- Fat: 7g
- Carbs: 29g
- Protein: 3g
- Fiber: 5g

39. Wild Rice and Mushroom Soup

Ingredients:

- 1 teaspoon of olive oil
- 1 diced onion
- 2 minced carrots,
- 2 minced celery stalks,
- 3 mugs of sliced mushrooms,
- 1 mug of rinsed wild rice,
- 6 mugs of vegetable broth.
- 1 tablespoon of thyme.
- Salt and pepper.
- 1/2 mug of heavy cream (optional for vegan, forget or substitute almond milk)

Instructions:

1. In a large pot, toast the olive oil over medium heat.

2. Cook the onion, carrots, celery, and mushrooms for about 10 minutes, or until softened.

3. Mix the wild rice, vegetable broth, and thyme.

4. Bring to a boil, then reduce the heat, cover and cook until rice is cooked, about 45 minutes.

5. Season with salt and pepper.

6. Stir in the heavy cream and heat until completely combined, if using.

7. Serve hot.

Preparation time: 15 minutes
Cooking time: 55 minutes

Nutritional value (per serving):

- Calories (without cream): 220
- Fat: 5g
- Carbs: 39g
- Protein: 8g
- Fiber: 4g

40. Vegetable Curry

Ingredients:

- 1 teaspoon of vegetable oil
- 1 onion, diced
- 2 garlic cloves, diced
- 1 teaspoon of curry powder.
- 1 tablespoon of ground turmeric.
- 1 can (14 ounces) of Coconut Milk

- 2 mugs of veggie broth.
- 2 potatoes, cubed
- 1 carrot, sliced
- 1 bell pepper, minced
- 1 mug frozen peas.
- Salt
- Fresh cilantro, diced (to garnish)

Instructions:

1. In a big pot, toast the oil over medium heat.

2. Cook for 5 minutes, or until the onion and garlic are softened.

3. Add curry powder and turmeric, and simmer for 1 minute.

4. Mix the coconut milk, vegetable broth, potatoes, and carrots.

5. Bring to a boil, then reduce heat and simmer for 20 minutes, or until the vegetables are cooked.

6. Add the bell pepper and peas, and simmer for another 5 minutes.

7. Season with salt.

8. Sprinkle with cilantro and serve.

Preparation time: 15 minutes

Cooking time: 30 minutes

Nutritional value (per serving):

- Calories: 250
- Fat: 14g
- Carbs: 28g
- Protein: 5g
- Fiber: 6g

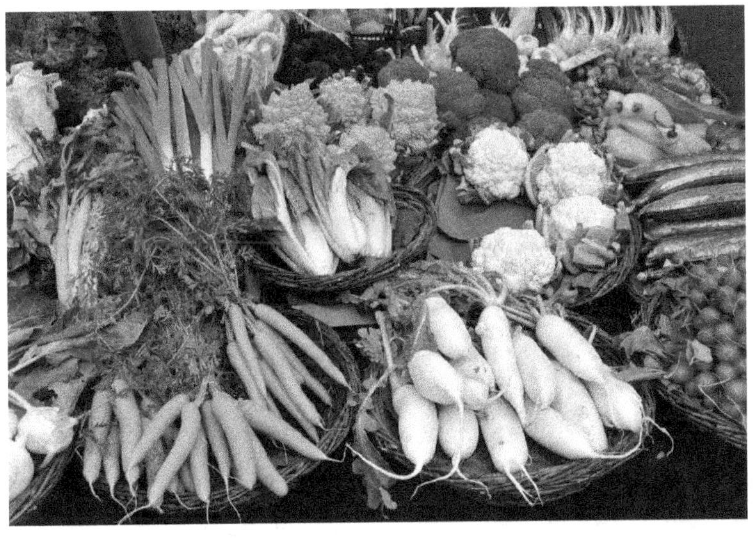

Kidney-Friendly Main Dishes

41. Baked Salmon with Lemon-Dill Sauce

Ingredients:

- 4 salmon filets.
- 2 teaspoons of olive oil.
- 1 lemon, sliced
- Salt and pepper

For lemon and dill sauce:

- 1/2 mug of greek yogurt.
- 2 teaspoons of fresh dill, chopped
- Juice from 1 lemon
- Salt and pepper to taste.

Instructions:

1. Preheat the oven to 375°F (190°C).

2. Place the salmon filets on a baking tray lined with parchment paper.

3. Drizzle olive oil over the fish and season with salt and pepper. Arrange the lemon slices on top.

4. Bake for 15-20 minutes, or until the salmon flaked easily with a fork.

5. While the salmon bakes, make the sauce by combining Greek yogurt, fresh dill, lemon juice, salt, and pepper.

6. Serve cooked fish with lemon-dill sauce on top.

Preparation time: 10 minutes.
Cooking time: 15-20 minutes.

Nutritional value (per serving):

- Calories: 300
- Fat: 18g
- Carbs: 2g
- Protein. 32g
- Fber. 1g

42. Turkey and Vegetable Stir-Fry

Ingredients:

- 1 pound of ground turkey.
- 2 teaspoons of vegetable oil.
- 1 onion, chopped
- 2 garlic cloves, minced
- 1 bell pepper, sliced

- 1 zucchini, sliced
- 1 mug of broccoli florets.
- 1/4 mug of soy sauce.
- 1 spoonful honey.
- 1 teaspoon of grated ginger.
- Salt and pepper
- Cooked rice or noodles are optional when serving.

Instructions:

1. In a large skillet, heat the vegetable oil over a medium heat.

2. Add the ground turkey and heat until browned, breaking it up with a spoon as you go.

3. Remove the turkey from the skillet and set it aside.

4. In the same skillet, cook the onion and garlic for 2 minutes.

5. Combine the bell peppers, zucchini, and broccoli. Stir-fry the vegetables for at least 5 minutes or until set.

6. Return cooked turkey to the skillet.

7. In a small bowl, mix together the soy sauce, honey, ginger, salt, and pepper.

8. Pour over the turkey and vegetables. Cook for 2–3 minutes, or until well cooked.

9. Serve hot with cooked rice or noodles, if preferred.

Preparation time: 15 minutes.
Cooking time: 20 minutes.

Nutritional value (per Serving):

- Calories: 300
- Fat: 15g
- Carbs: 20g
- Protein: 26g
- Fiber: 4g

43. Lemon-Herbal Grilled Chicken

Ingredients:

- 4 boneless, skinless chicken breasts.
- 2 teaspoons of olive oil.
- 2 garlic cloves, minced
- Juice from 1 lemon zest
- 1 tablespoon of fresh thyme, chopped
- Salt and pepper

Instructions:

1. In a mixing bowl, combine olive oil, minced garlic, lemon zest, lemon juice, fresh thyme, salt, and pepper to make a marinade.

2. Put the chicken breasts in a resealable plastic bag or shallow plate.

3. Pour the marinade over the chicken and seal the bag or cover the dish.

4. Refrigerate for at least 30 minutes, or up to two hours.

5. Preheat the grill to medium-high heat and lightly oil the grates.

6. Remove the chicken from the marinade and grill for 6-7 minutes per side, or until fully cooked.

7. Serve hot.

Preparation time: 10 minutes (including marinating).
Cooking time: 14 minutes.

Nutritional Value (per serving):

- Calories: 220
- Fat: 10g
- Carbs: 2g
- Protein: 30g

- Fiber: 0g

44. Vegetable and Tofu Stir-fry

Ingredients:

- 1 block (14 oz) of tofu, diced
- 2 teaspoons of vegetable oil.
- 2 garlic cloves, minced
- 1 bell pepper, sliced
- 1 mug of broccoli florets.
- 1 mug of snap peas.
- 1 carrot cut
- 1/4 mug of soy sauce.
- 1 spoonful honey.
- 1 teaspoon of grated ginger.
- Salt and pepper
- Cooked rice or noodles are optional when serving.

Instructions:

1. Press the tofu to remove any extra water, then cut it into cubes.

2. In a large skillet, heat the vegetable oil over a medium heat. Cook the tofu cubes until golden brown on all sides.

3. Remove the tofu from the skillet and set aside.

4. In the same skillet, sauté the minced garlic for 1 minute.

5. Combine the bell peppers, broccoli, snap peas, and carrots.

6. Stir-fry the vegetables for about 5 minutes, or until tender and crispy.

7. Return cooked tofu to the skillet.

8. In a small bowl, mix together the soy sauce, honey, ginger, salt, and pepper. Pour over the tofu and veggies.

9. Cook for 2–3 minutes, or until well cooked.

10. Serve hot with cooked rice or noodles, if preferred.

Preparation time: 20 minutes.
Cooking time: 15 minutes.

Nutritional Value (per serving):

- Calories: 280
- Fat: 14g
- Carbs: 22g
- Protein: 18g
- Fiber: 4g

45. Eggplant Parmesan

Ingredients:

- 2 eggplants sliced into rounds.
- 2 mugs of breadcrumbs.
- 2 mugs of marinara sauce.
- 2 mugs of shredded mozzarella cheese.
- 1/2 mugs of grated Parmesan cheese.
- 2 eggs, beaten
- 2 teaspoons of olive oil.
- Salt and pepper
- Fresh basil leaves (for garnish)

Instructions:

1. Preheat the oven to 375°F (190°C).

2. In a small plate, place the beaten eggs. In another shallow dish, place the breadcrumbs.

3. Dip eggplant slices into beaten eggs, letting the excess drip off, and then coat with breadcrumbs.

4. Place on a baking sheet.

5. Drizzle olive oil over the breaded eggplant slices. Bake for 20–25 minutes, or until golden brown and tender.

6. In a baking dish, spread a thin layer of marinara.

7. Layer half of the baked eggplant slices, followed by more sauce, mozzarella cheese, and Parmesan cheese. Repeat the layers.

8. Bake for an additional 20 minutes, or until the cheese has melted and browned.

9. Garnish with fresh basil and serve hot.

Preparation time: 20 minutes
Cooking time: 45 minutes.

Nutritional Value (per serving):

- Calories: 380
- Fat: 17g
- Carbs: 41g
- Protein: 18g
- Fiber: 10g

46. Quinoa and Black Beans Stuffed Peppers

Ingredients:

- 4 bell peppers of any color
- 1 mug of quinoa, washed
- 2 mugs of vegetable broth.

- 1 can (15 ounces) of black beans, dried and rinsed
- 1 mug of corn kernels (fresh, frozen, or canned).
- 1 mug of diced tomatoes.
- 1 tablespoon of chili powder.
- 1/2 tablespoon of cumin.
- Salt and pepper.
- 1 mug of shredded cheddar cheese (optional).

Instructions:

1. Heat the oven to 375 °F (190 °C).

2. Cut off the bell pepper tops and remove the seeds and membranes. Set away.

3. In a saucepan, mix the quinoa and the vegetable broth.

4. Bring to a boil, then reduce the heat, cover and simmer for at least 15 minutes or until the quinoa is cooked.

5. In a large mixing coliseum, add the cooked quinoa, black beans, corn, minced tomatoes, chili powder, cumin, salt and pepper.

6. Cover the bell peppers with the mixture of quinoa and black beans.

7. Put the stuffed peppers in a baking dish and cover with aluminum foil.

8. Bake for about 25-30 minutes or until the peppers have softened.

9. Put shredded cheddar cheese on top and bake for another 5 minutes or until melted, If needed.

10. Serve hot.

Preparation time: 15 minutes
Cooking time: 45 minutes

Nutritional value (per serving):

- Calories: 280
- Fat: 4g
- Carbs: 50g
- Protein: 12g
- Fiber: 9g

47. Roasted Vegetable and Chickpea Bowl

Ingredients:

- 2 mugs of mixed vegetables (i.e cherry tomatoes, zucchini, and bell peppers)
- 1 can (15 oz) of drained and washed chickpeas.
- 2 teaspoons of olive oil

- 1 tablespoon of paprika.
- 1/2 tablespoon of cumin.
- Salt and pepper.
- Cooked quinoa or rice is optional for serving.
- Tahini dressing (optional to mizzle).

Instructions:

1. Preheat the oven to 425 °F(220 °C).

2. In a large mixing coliseum, add the vegetables, chickpeas, olive oil, paprika, cumin, salt and pepper.

3. Spread the mixture inversely across a baking dish.

4. Roast the vegetables in the oven for at least 20-25 minutes, until soft and gently browned.

5. Serve over cooked quinoa or rice, with tahini dressing if needed.

Preparation time: 10 minutes
Cooking time: 25 minutes

Nutritional value (per serving, without quinoa and dressing):

- Calories: 200
- Fat: 7g

- Carbs: 30g
- Protein: 8g
- Fiber: 8g

48. Baked Cod with Tomato and Olive Relish

Ingredients:

- 4 cod fillets.
- 2 teaspoons of olive oil
- 2 garlic cloves, diced
- 1 can (14.5 oz), of diced tomatoes drained
- 1/2 mug of Kalamata olives, pitted and diced
- 2 teaspoons of fresh basil, diced
- Salt and pepper.
- Lemon wedges (for garnish).

Instructions

1. Heat the oven to 375 °F (190 °C).

2. Put the cod fillets on a roasting tray.

3. In a coliseum, mix the olive oil, garlic, tomatoes, olives, basil, salt and pepper.

4. Spread the tomato and olive relish on the cod fillets.

5. Use aluminum foil to cover the baking dish.

6. Bake for 20-25 minutes or until the fish is completely cooked and easily flaked.

7. Serve hot with lemon wedges for garnish.

Preparation time: 10 minutes
Cooking time: 25 minutes

Nutritional value (per serving):

- Calories: 200
- Fat: 9g
- Carbs: 8g
- Protein: 28g
- Fiber: 2g

49. Spaghetti Squash Primavera

Ingredients:

- 1 spaghetti squash.
- 1 teaspoon of olive oil
- 1 onion, diced
- 2 garlic cloves, diced
- 1 mug of cherry tomatoes, halved
- 1 mug of broccoli florets.

- 1 mug of bell peppers, sliced
- 1/2 mug of grated Parmesan rubbish.
- Fresh basil leaves (for garnish)
- Salt and pepper.

Instructions:

1. Heat the oven to 375 °F (190 °C).

2. Remove the seeds and cut the spaghetti squash in half along its length.

3. Place the squash halves, cut side down, on a baking sheet.

4. Bake for 30-40 minutes or until the squash is tender and scrapeable with a chopstick.

5. While the squash bakes, heat the olive oil in a skillet over a medium heat.

6. Cook the onion and garlic until softened for at least about 5 minutes.

7. Mix the cherry tomatoes, broccoli, and bell pepper.

8. Cook for at least 5 minutes or until the vegetables are tender and crunchy.

9. Scrape the flesh of the cooked spaghetti squash with a chopstick to form "noodles."

10. Mix the squash "noodles" with the cooked vegetables and grated Parmesan. Season with salt and pepper.

11. Garnish with fresh basil and serve hot.

Preparation time: 10 minutes (including baking time for squash).
Cooking time: 15 minutes

Nutritional value (per serving):

- Calories: 180
- Fat: 9g
- Carbs: 21g
- Protein: 7g
- Fiber: 5g

50. Cauliflower Rice Bowl

Ingredients:

- 1 head of cauliflower, cut into florets.
- 2 teaspoons of olive oil
- 1 onion, diced
- 2 garlic cloves, diced

- 1 mug of diced bell peppers
- 1 mug of diced cucumber.
- 1/2 mug of diced tomatoes.
- 1/4 mug of freshly diced parsley.
- 1/4 mug of crumbled feta (optional).
- Juice from 1 lemon
- Salt and pepper.
- Hummus (optional, for serving)

Instructions

1. Put the cauliflower florets in a food processor and palpitation until they act rice or couscous.

2. In a large skillet, heat the olive oil over a medium heat.

3. Cook the diced onion and garlic until softened for at least about 5 minutes.

4. Cook cauliflower "rice" for 5-7 minutes, tossing occasionally, until tender and gently browned.

5. Remove from heat and let cool slightly.

6. In a coliseum, mix the cooked cauliflower "rice," minced bell peppers, cucumber, tomatoes, fresh parsley, and a crumbled feta cheese (if using).

7. Mizzle lemon juice over the mixture and season with salt and pepper.

8. Serve in a coliseum with a nugget of hummus, if needed.

Preparation time: 15 minutes
Cooking time: 15 minutes

Nutritional value (per serving, without feta rubbish and hummus)

- Calories: 120
- Fat: 7g
- Carbs: 14g
- Protein: 4g
- Fiber: 5g

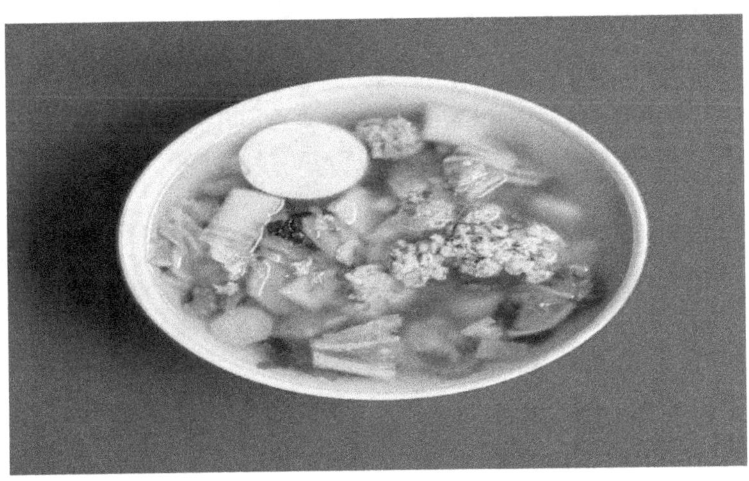

Sides and Snacks

51. Zucchini Fritters

Ingredients:

- 2 medium zucchini, grated
- 1/2 tablespoon salt
- 1/4 mug shredded Parmesan cheese
- 1/4 mug breadcrumbs.
- 1/4 mug diced fresh sauces (like parsley or dill)
- 1/4 mug diced green onions.
- 1 egg, beaten
- 2 soupspoons olive oil (for frying).
- Dip with Greek yogurt or sour cream (optional).

Instructions:

1. Place the shredded zucchini in a strainer, sprinkle with salt, and let it drain for 10 minutes to remove excess moisture.

2. Squeeze the zucchini to extract as much juice as possible.

3. In a mixing dish, mix the grated zucchini, Parmesan cheese, breadcrumbs, diced sauces, green onions, and beaten eggs. Mix thoroughly.

4. In a medium- sized skillet, heat the olive oil.

5. Scoop spoonfuls of the zucchini mixture into the skillet and flatten with a spatula.

6. Cook until golden brown on both sides for about 3-4 minutes each.

7. Remove from the skillet and allow to drain on paper towels.

8. Serve hot with Greek yogurt or sour cream for dipping, if using.

Preparation time: 20 minutes
Cooking time: 8 minutes

Nutritional value (per serving, without dipping sauce):

- Calories: 80
- Fat: 4g
- Carbs: 8g
- Protein: 3g
- Fiber: 1g

52. Homemade Hummus

Ingredients:

- 1 can (15 oz) of drained and washed chickpeas.
- 3 soupspoons tahini.
- 2 garlic cloves, diced
- Juice from 1 lemon
- 2 teaspoons olive oil
- 1/2 tablespoon cumin.
- Salt and pepper
- Water (as demanded for proper thickness).
- Garnish with paprika and olive oil (optional).

Instructions:

1. In a food processor, mix chickpeas, tahini, diced garlic, lemon juice, olive oil, cumin, salt and pepper.

2. Mix until smooth, scraping down the sides of the coliseum as demanded.

3. Add water, one teaspoon at a time, If the hummus is too thick.

4. Taste and adjust seasonings as demanded.

5. Transfer to a serving coliseum.

6. Mizzle with olive oil and sprinkle with paprika for garnish, If needed.

7. Serve with pita bread, crackers, or vegetable sticks.

Preparation time: 10 minutes

Cooking time: 0 minutes

Nutritive value per serving (without garnish):

- Calories: 90
- Fat: 6g
- Carbs: 8g
- Protein: 3g
- Fiber: 2g

53. Crispy Baked Kale Chips

Ingredients:

- 1 bunch kale, stems removed and leaves torn into bite- sized pieces.
- 1 teaspoon olive oil
- Salt and pepper
- Optional additions (i.e nutritive yeast and garlic powder)

Instructions:

1. Preheat the oven to 350 °F/ 175 °C.

2. In a large coliseum, toss the kale with olive oil, salt, pepper and any other needed additions.

3. Arrange the kale in a single layer on a baking sheet.

4. Baked for 10-15 minutes or until kale is crisp and smoothly browned. Observe them closely to prevent them from burning.

5. Remove from the oven and let it cool before serving.

Preparation time: 10 minutes
Cooking time: 10- 15 minutes

Nutritional value (per Serving):

- Calories: 50
- Fat: 4g
- Carbs: 6g
- Protein: 2g
- Fiber: 2g

54. Roasted Sweet Potato Wedges

Ingredients:

- 2 big sweet potatoes, hulled and cut into wedges
- 2 teaspoons of olive oil
- 1 tablespoon of paprika.
- 1/2 tablespoon cayenne pepper (adjust to taste).
- Salt and pepper

- Fresh parsley (for garnish, optional)

Instructions:

1. Preheat the oven to 425 °F (220 °C).

2. In a large mixing coliseum, toss sweet potato wedges with olive oil, paprika, cayenne pepper, salt and pepper.

3. Place the sweet potato wedges in a single layer on a baking sheet.

4. Roast the wedges for at least 25- 30 minutes, flipping half through, until they're soft and slightly crisp.

5. Serve hot and sprinkle with fresh parsley if needed.

Preparation time: 10 minutes
Cooking time: 25-30 minutes

Nutritional value (per Serving):

- Calories: 120
- Fat: 5g
- Carbs: 19g
- Protein: 2g
- Fiber: 3g

55. Guacamole and Vegetable Sticks

Ingredients:

- 3 ripe avocados, peeled and pitted
- 1 tomato, minced.
- 1/4 mug minced red onion.
- 2 garlic cloves, diced
- Juice from 1 lime
- Salt and pepper
- Carrot sticks, cucumber slices, bell pepper strips (for dip).

Instructions:

1. Mash the avocados in a coliseum with a fork until smooth completely.

2. Mix the minced tomato, red onion, diced garlic, lime juice, salt and pepper. Mix thoroughly.

3. Taste and adjust the seasonings as demanded.

4. Dip in carrot sticks, cucumber slices, and bell pepper strips.

Preparation time: 15 minutes
Cooking time: 0 minutes

Nutritional value (per serving, without dipping vegetables):

- Calories: 180
- Fat: 15g
- Carbs: 12g
- Protein: 3g
- Fiber: 7g

56. Greek Yogurt and Berry Parfait

Ingredients:

- 1 mug Greek yogurt.
- 1/2 mug mixed berries (i.e strawberries, blueberries and snorts) 1/4 mug granola.
- Honey is optional for spraying.

Instructions:

1. In a glass or dish, stir the Greek yogurt, mixed berries and granola.

2. Repeat the layers as needed.

3. Mizzle with honey if you want it sweeter.

4. Serve immediately.

Preparation time: 5 minute
Cooking time: 0 minutes

Nutritional value per serving (without honey):

- Calories: 250
- Fat: 7g
- Carbs: 31g
- Protein: 16g
- Fiber: 3g

57. Trail mix

Ingredients:

- 1/2 mug almonds.
- 1/2 mug cashews.
- 1/2 mug dried cranberries.
- 1/4 mug of dark chocolate chips.
- 1/4 mug pumpkin seeds.
- 1/4 mug raisins.

Instructions:

1. In a coliseum, mix all the ingredients.

2. Store in a watertight vessel for a accessible on-the-go snack.

Preparation time: 5 minutes
Cooking time: 0 minute

Nutritive value (per Serving):

- Calories: 250
- Fat: 15g
- Carbs: 24g
- Protein: 5g
- Fiber: 4g

58. Cucumber Slices with Tzatziki.

Ingredients:

1 cucumber, sliced
1/2 mug tzatziki sauce (store bought or homemade).

Instructions:

1. Place the cucumber slices on a dish.

2. Serve with tzatziki sauce for dipping.

Preparation time: 5 minutes
Cooking time: 0 minute

Nutritional value (per Serving):

- Calories: 80
- Fat: 6g
- Carbs: 6g
- Protein: 2g
- Fiber: 1g

59. Almond and Date Energy Balls

Ingredients:

- 1 mug almonds.
- 1 mug pitted dates.
- 1/4 mug cocoa powder.
- 1/4 mug almond butter.
- 1/4 mug honey.
- 1/2 teaspoon of vanilla excerpt.
- A pinch of salt.
- Rolling with shredded coconut or diced almonds is optional.

Instructions:

1. Place almonds in a food processor and pulse until coarsely smashed.

2. Mix pitted dates, cocoa powder, almond butter, honey, vanilla substance, and a pinch of salt in a food processor.

3. Blend the constituents until they produce a sticky dough.

4. Scoop out small portions of the mixture and form into balls.

5. To add texture, fleece the energy balls with shredded coconut or diced almonds.

6. Place the energy balls in a watertight vessel and chill until solidified.

7. Enjoy this quick and healthy snack.

Preparation time: 15 minutes
Cooking time: 0 minute

Nutritional value (per serving, without optional coatings):

- Calories: 120
- Fat: 6g
- Carbs: 16g
- Protein: 3g
- Fiber: 3g

60. Mixed Berry Smoothie Bowl

Ingredients:

- 1 mug mixed berries (i.e strawberries, blueberries, and snorts)
- 1/2 mug greek yogurt.
- 1/4 mug rolled oats.
- 1 spoonful honey.
- Fresh berries, sliced banana, and granola (topping, optional).

Instructions:

1. In a blender, combine mixed berries, Greek yogurt, rolled oats and honey.

2. Mix until smooth completely.

3. Pour the smoothie into a coliseum.

4. Fresh berries, sliced bananas, and granola are also optional additions.

5. Serve immediately.

Preparation time: 5 minutes
Cooking time: 0 minute

Nutritive value per serving (without condiments):

- Calories: 250
- Fat: 4g

- Carbs: 40g
- Protein: 14g
- Fiber: 5g

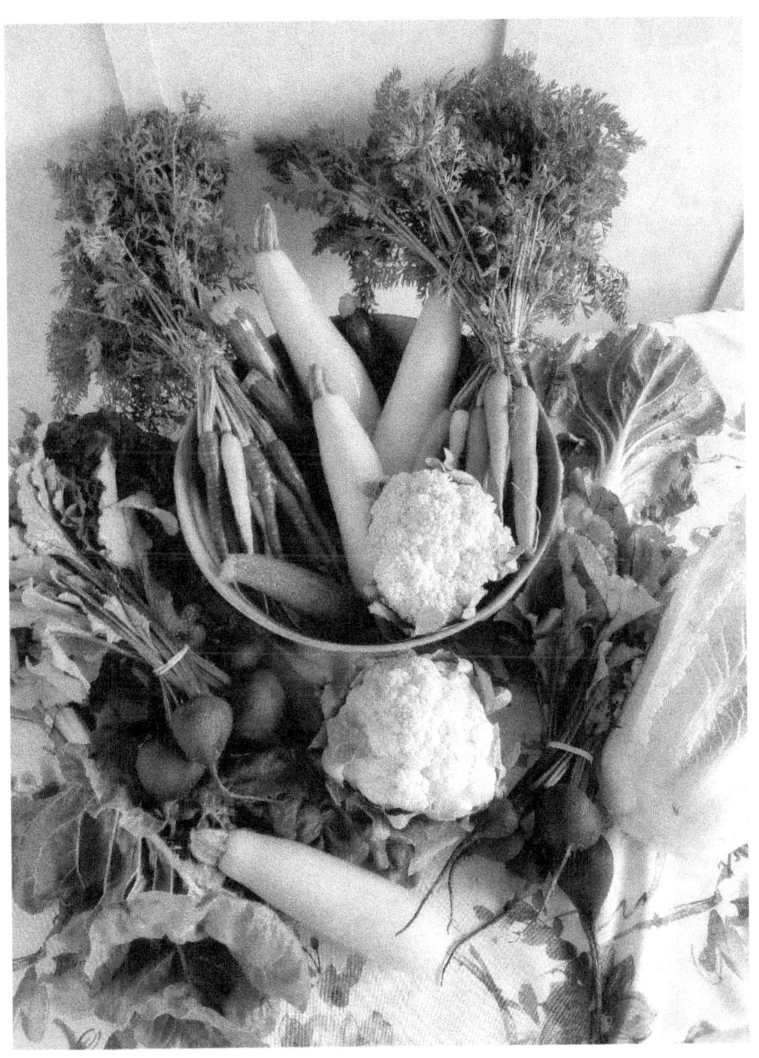

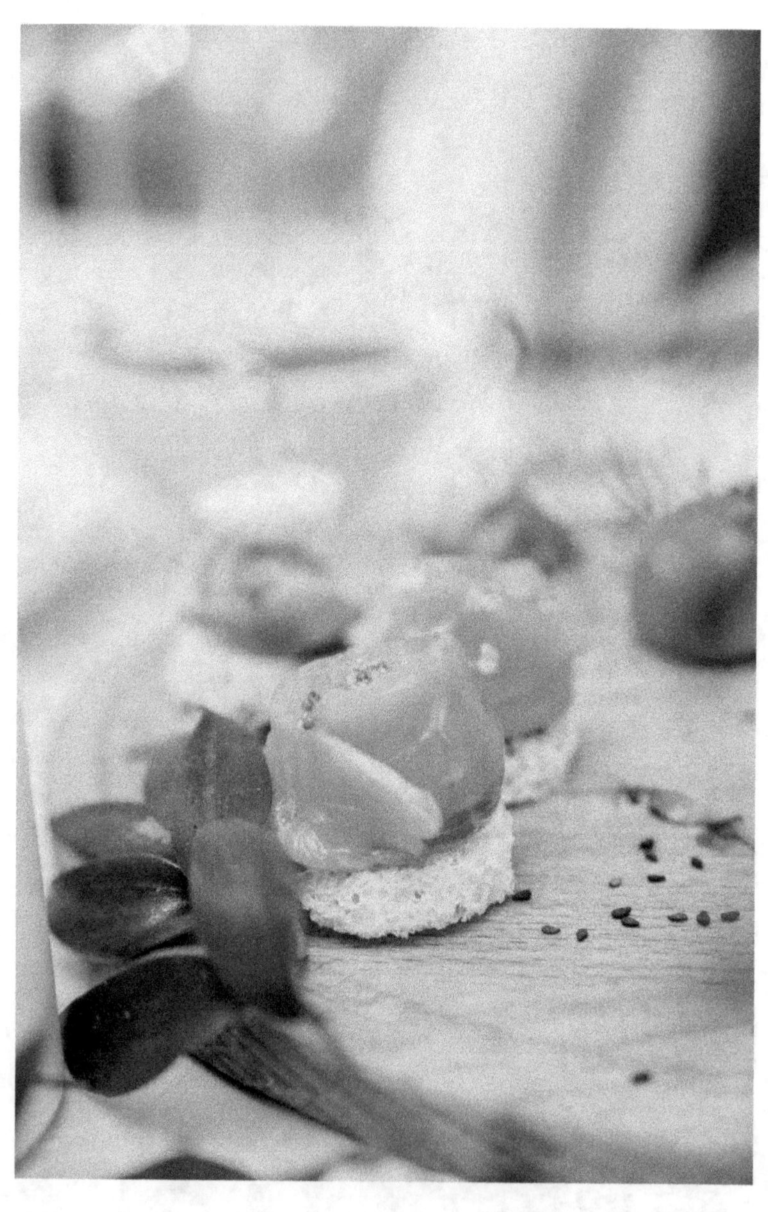

CHAPTER 6: HERBAL SUPPLEMENTS FOR KIDNEY HEALTH

This chapter looks at a variety of natural therapies and substances that can help with kidney health. We'll look at individual herbs with renal advantages, supplements that help with kidney function, and crucial lifestyle factors to keep your kidneys healthy.

Beneficial Herbs for Kidney Cleaning

Herbs have been used for millennia in traditional medicine to promote kidney health. Listed below are some of the most effective:

1. Dandelion Root: Acts as a natural diuretic, assisting the kidneys in eliminating extra salt and water. Dandelion root is also beneficial in cleansing the kidneys and liver.

2. Stinging Nettle: This herb has long been utilized for its anti-inflammatory characteristics and capacity to help eliminate toxins from the body, including the kidneys. It also contains antioxidants, which protect the kidneys from harm.

3. Parsley: Known for its diuretic characteristics, parsley can assist the kidneys clear waste while also controlling blood pressure, which is an important element in kidney health.

4. Ginger can help cleanse the body by promoting digestion, circulation, and sweating. Its natural cleaning effects improve renal function.

5. Turmeric: This herb has anti-inflammatory qualities. Chronic inflammation can compromise kidney health, but turmeric can help protect the kidneys.

6. Cranberries are commonly used to treat urinary tract infections, but they can also assist preserve kidney health by preventing bacteria from adhering to the bladder and urinary system walls.

Supplements that Improve Kidney Function

Supplements can help support kidney health.

1. Omega-3 fatty acids are vital for decreasing inflammation and have been demonstrated to protect the kidneys.

2. Probiotics support a healthy gut flora, which has been associated with improved kidney function and a lower risk of renal disease.

3. Magnesium: Adequate magnesium levels reduce the production of kidney stones.

4. Vitamin B6 decreases the production of calcium oxalate, which is a major contributor to kidney stones.

5. Potassium citrate is useful for alkalizing urine and avoiding stone formation.

Dos and Don'ts for Kidney Health

Maintaining kidney health entails more than simply taking herbs and vitamins. Here are some important do's and don'ts.

1. Maintain proper kidney function by staying hydrated.

2. Monitor your blood pressure and sugar levels: High levels might put a strain on your kidneys.

3. Consume a Balanced Diet: A diet high in fruits, vegetables, whole grains, and lean proteins can benefit kidney function.

4. Avoid: Overuse. Painkillers: Nonsteroidal anti-inflammatory medications (NSAIDs) can be harmful to the kidneys.

5. Consume Excess Protein: A high protein intake might strain the kidneys.

6. Smoking or drinking excessively can compromise kidney function and cause kidney injury.

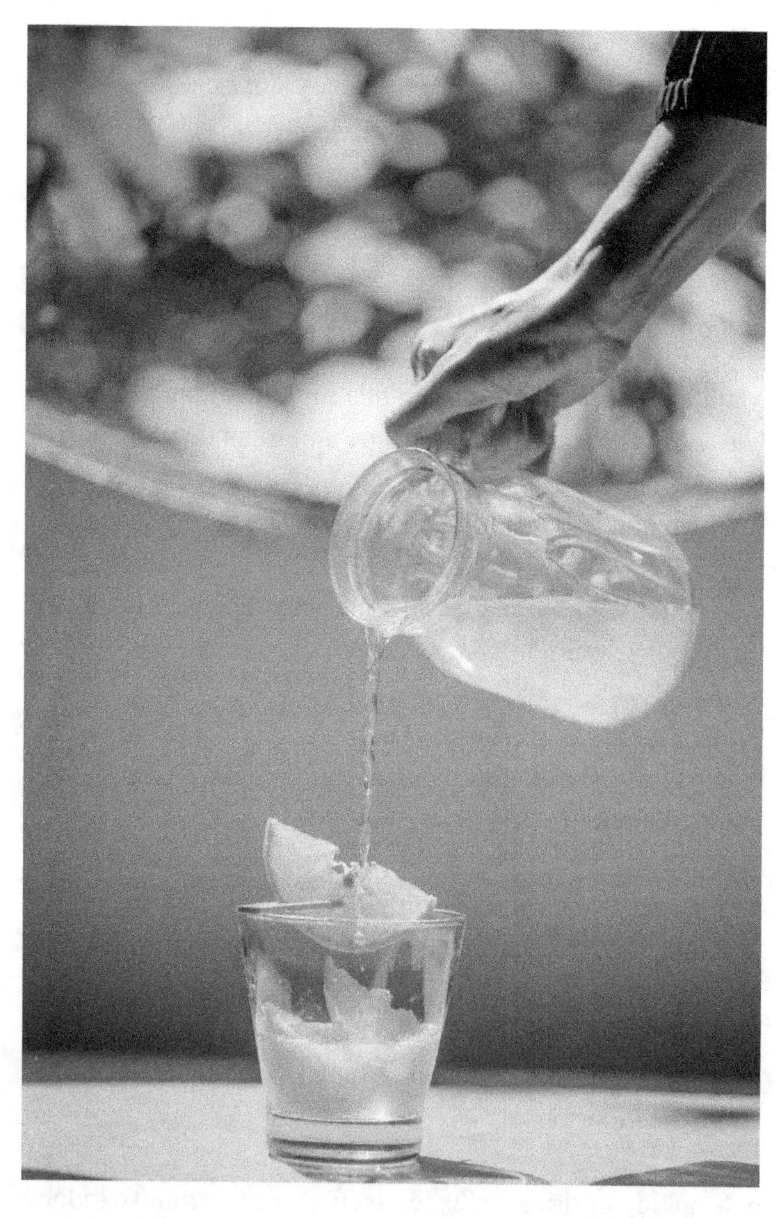

CHAPTER 7: 7-DAY AND 14-DAY DETOX PLAN

This chapter contains systematic detox methods designed to improve kidney health. These regimens are intended to eliminate toxins, promote renal function, and enhance general health.

We'll go over a 7-day kidney cleanse plan for a quick reset, as well as a longer 14-day detox. In addition, we offer ideas to assist you stay on track during these detox times.

7-Day Kidney Cleansing Plan

Day 1-7:

- Morning: Begin each day with a warm glass of lemon water to improve digestion and initiate the detoxification process.

- Breakfast: Choose hydrating fruits such as watermelon or berries, along with a small serving of yogurt for bacteria.

- Lunch: Choose leafy green salads with herbs such as parsley and cilantro, which are recognized for their cleansing effects.

- Snacks: Choose kidney-friendly snacks such as apple slices or carrot sticks.

- Dinner: Serve lean protein (chicken or fish) with cruciferous vegetables such as broccoli or cauliflower.

- Hydration: Drink at least 8-10 glasses of water every day.

- Herbal Teas: Drink dandelion or nettle tea in the afternoon or evening.

The 14-Day Detox Plan

Week 1:

- Follow the 7-Day Kidney Cleansing Plan.

- Exercise: Light workouts such as walking or yoga might help with circulation and toxin clearance.

Week 2:

- Morning: Continue with the lemon water.

- Breakfast: Try oatmeal with chia seeds for fiber.

- Lunch and dinner: Begin introducing healthful grains such as quinoa and brown rice. Include kidney-friendly foods such as beets and sweet potatoes.

- Snacks: Nuts and seeds provide healthful fats.

- Hydration: Drink plenty of water; for added flavor, try cucumber or mint.

- Herbal Support: Continue drinking herbal teas, and try adding turmeric tea for its anti-inflammatory qualities.

Tips to Stay on Track

1. Preparation is key. To avoid eating on impulse, plan your meals and snacks ahead of time.

2. Mindful eating entails listening to your body's hunger and fullness cues. Eat attentively and enjoy your food.

3. Stay Hydrated: Carry a water bottle with you throughout the day to remind yourself to drink water on a regular basis.

4. Avoid Toxins: During the detox period, limit your intake of alcohol, caffeine, and processed meals.

5. Rest Adequately: Make sure you receive adequate sleep, as it is essential for detoxifying.

6. Track Your Progress: Keep a notebook to record how you feel every day. Take note of any changes in your energy levels, digestion, and overall well-being.

7. Seek Support: Tell your family and friends about your detox strategy to gain support and prevent temptations.

Following these detox strategies can help cleanse your kidneys and improve their function. It's critical to note that these plans should be used as a guideline, not as a replacement for medical advice.

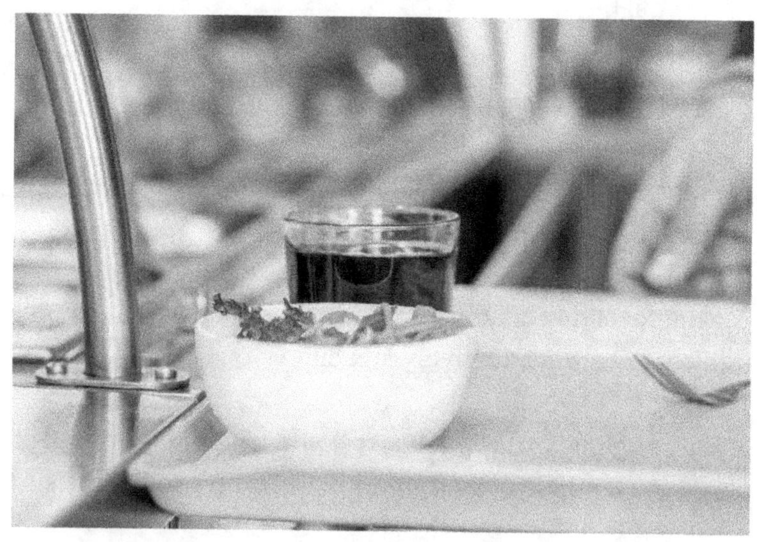

CHAPTER 8: BEYOND THE DIET A LIFESTYLE FOR HEALTHY KIDNEYS

This chapter focuses on the importance of lifestyle variables in kidney health. While food is important, other factors such as hydration, exercise, and stress management can also help the kidneys work properly.

This chapter digs into each of these topics, offering insights and practical strategies for incorporating them into your daily life.

Hydration and Kidney Health

Importance of Water:

- Water helps the kidneys remove waste and poisons from the blood. Adequate hydration can help prevent kidney stones and urinary tract infections.

- Recommendation: Aim for 8-10 glasses of water each day, while this may vary depending on individual needs, activity levels, and environment.

Monitor Hydration Levels:

- Learn to identify indicators of dehydration, such as dark urine, weariness, and dizziness.

- Tip: To stay hydrated, eat water-rich foods like fruits and vegetables.

Exercise and Kidney Function

Benefits of Physical Activity:

- Regular exercise promotes appropriate blood pressure and blood sugar levels, both of which are important for kidney health.

- It also aids in weight management and lowers the risk of kidney disease.

Recommended Types of Exercise

- Aerobic workouts such as walking, running, cycling, and swimming are very effective.

- Strength training is also an option, but your exercise plan should be tailored to your general health and fitness level.

Exercise Precautions:

Before beginning any new workout regimen, those with pre-existing renal difficulties should consult with their doctor.

Stress Management and Its Effect on Kidneys

Understanding the Connection:

Chronic stress can cause high blood pressure and bad lifestyle choices, compromising kidney health.

Effective Stress Management Techniques

- Mindfulness and meditation can assist to lower stress levels.

- Regular physical activity and hobbies can also help relieve stress.

Developing a Balanced Lifestyle:

- Get enough sleep, as sleep loss can worsen stress.

- Create a support network of friends, family, or support groups to assist you manage stress.

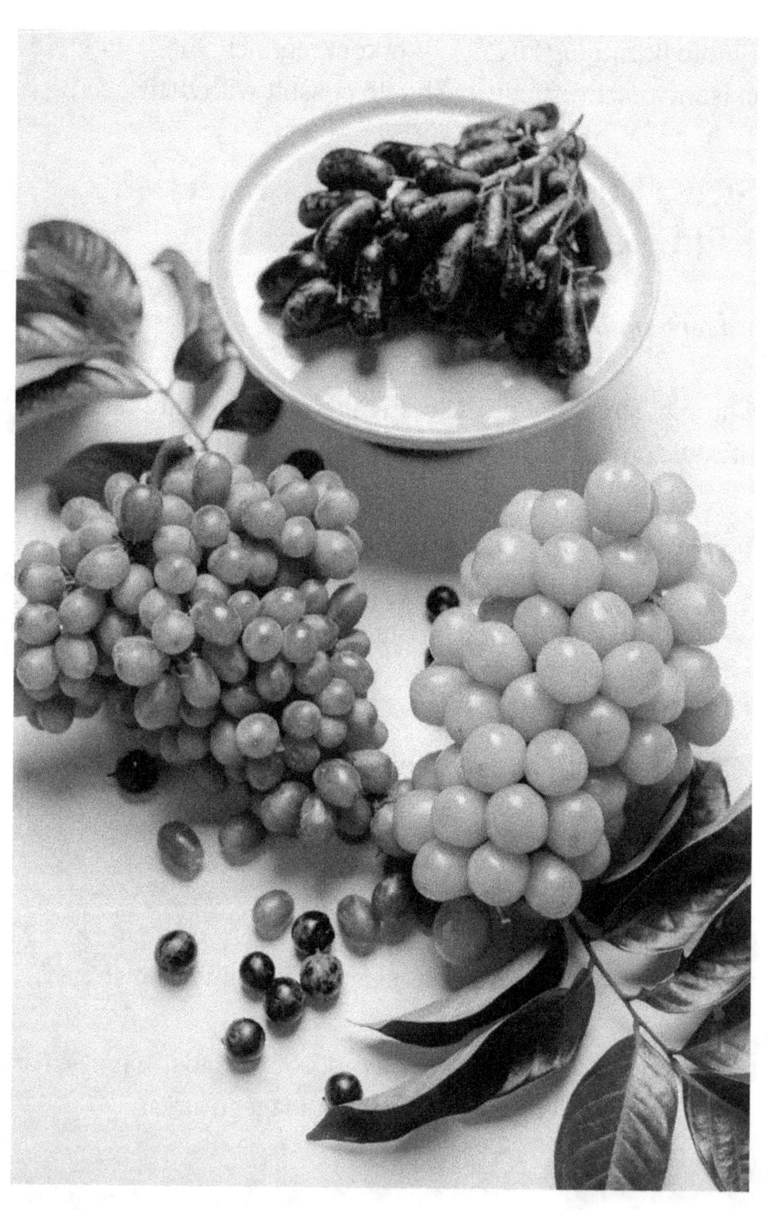

CONCLUSION

Throughout this book, we've looked at several aspects of kidney health, emphasizing the significance of taking a comprehensive approach to maintaining and increasing kidney function.

We discussed dietary changes, specific herbs and supplements that are beneficial to the kidneys, thorough detox regimens, and the importance of lifestyle aspects like hydration, exercise, and stress management.

In terms of nutrition, we saw how a well-balanced, kidney-friendly diet is critical to maintaining kidney health. We learnt about the benefits of various herbs and supplements for kidney function, as well as the significance of eating mindfully and avoiding items that can stress the kidneys.

The 7-day and 14-day detox regimens provided systematic approaches to resetting and rejuvenating kidney function, emphasizing the importance of gradual and consistent lifestyle modifications. These plans serve not only as a detoxifying procedure, but also as a launch for long-term kidney-friendly habits.

Furthermore, we emphasized the need of hydration, regular physical activity, and appropriate stress management in maintaining kidney function. Adequate water intake ensures that the kidneys operate properly, exercise promotes overall health and renal efficiency, and stress management is critical in preventing high blood pressure and other risk factors for kidney disease.

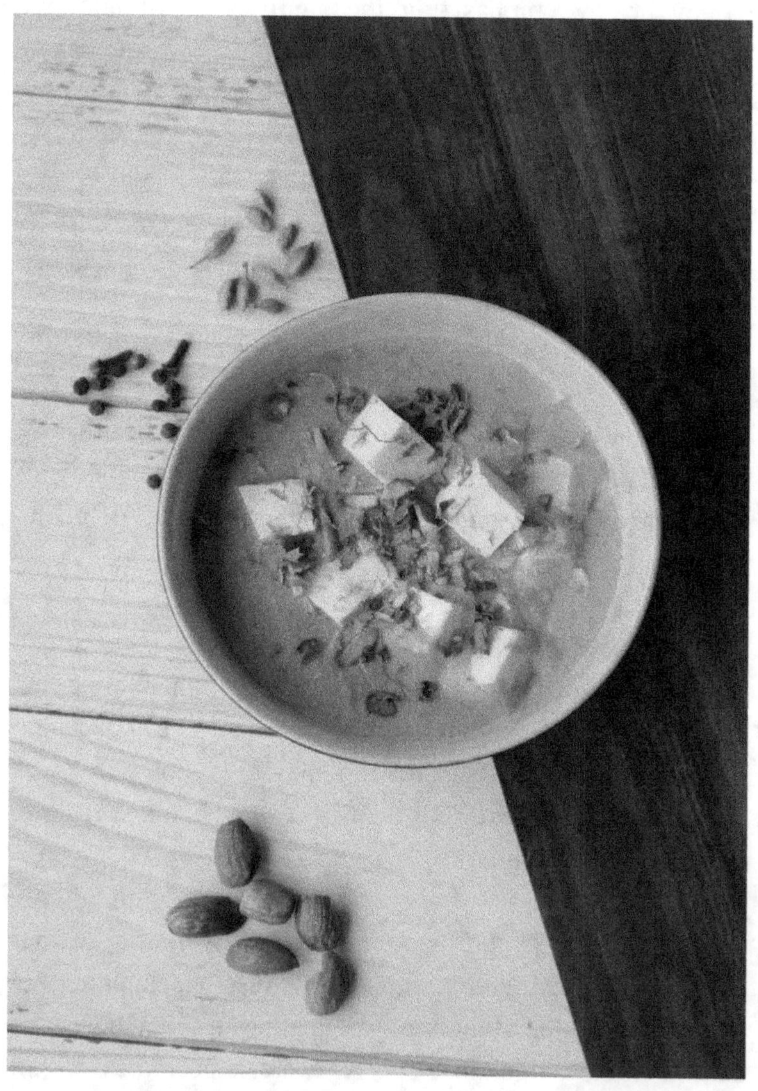

GLOSSARY

Glossary of Kidney Health Guide

1. Antioxidants: are substances that can prevent or reduce damage to cells caused by free radicals, hence lowering oxidative stress. Frequently found in fruits and vegetables.

2. Chronic Kidney Disease (CKD): is a long-term illness in which the kidneys do not function properly. CKD can lead to end-stage renal disease in extreme situations.

3. Detoxification (detox): is the process of eliminating hazardous substances or attributes. In the context of renal health, it refers to dietary and lifestyle habits that help to cleanse the kidneys.

4. Diuretic: A substance that causes diuresis, or the increased output of urine. Certain foods and beverages have diuretic characteristics that help to cleanse the kidneys.

5. Electrolytes: are minerals in your body that carry an electric charge and are necessary for numerous human functions. Common electrolytes include sodium, potassium, and magnesium.

6. Glomerular Filtration Rate (GFR): A test that determines how effectively the kidneys filter blood. It is a key indication of renal function.

7. Hemodialysis: is a medical therapy that removes waste products and extra fluid from the blood when the kidneys are not functioning properly.

8. Nephrologists: are doctors who specialize in kidney care and illness treatment.

9. Probiotics: Live bacteria and yeasts that are beneficial to your health, particularly your digestive system. They are commonly known as "good" or "helpful" bacteria.

10. Proteinuria: Abnormal protein levels in the urine, which can indicate kidney disease.

11. Renal: Refers to the kidneys.

12. Renal Diet: A diet recommended for persons who have kidney disease. The diet typically minimizes nutrients such as phosphorus, potassium, and sodium.

13. Urinary Tract Infection (UTI): is an infection of any component of the urinary system, such as the kidneys, bladder, or urethra.

14. Urologist: A doctor who specializes in illnesses of the urinary tract and male reproductive system.

INDEX

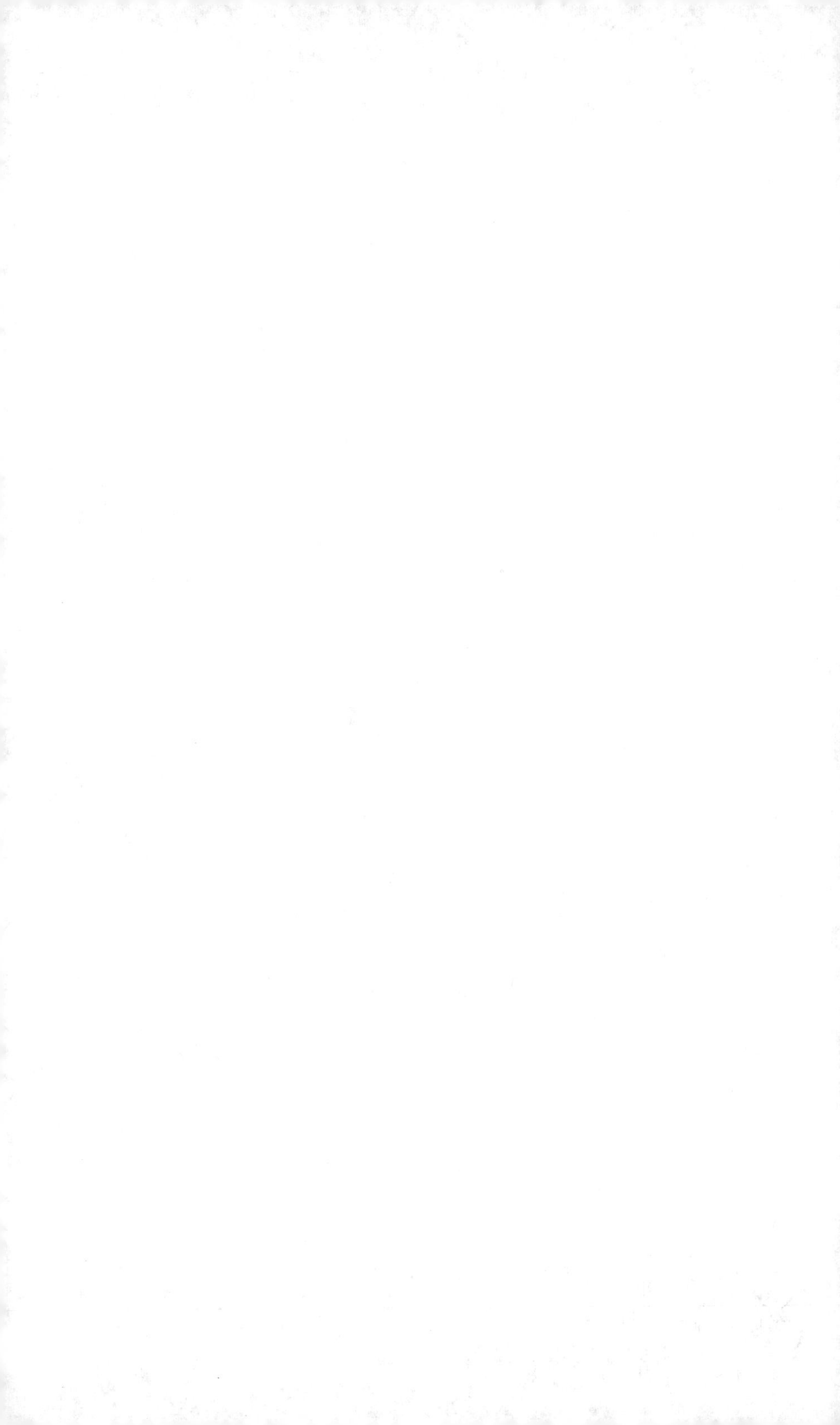